The
TAO
of
WING CHUN

*The History and Principles of China's
Most Explosive Martial Art*

Danny Xuan

and

John Little

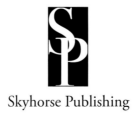

Skyhorse Publishing

Skyhorse Publishing books may be purchased in bulk at special discounts for sales promotion, corporate gifts, fund-raising, or educational purposes. Special editions can also be created to specifications. For details, contact the Special Sales Department, Skyhorse Publishing, 307 West 36th Street, 11th Floor, New York, NY 10018 or info@skyhorsepublishing.com.

Skyhorse® and Skyhorse Publishing® are registered trademarks of Skyhorse Publishing, Inc.®, a Delaware corporation.

Visit our website at www.skyhorsepublishing.com.

10 9 8 7 6 5 4 3 2

Library of Congress Cataloging-in-Publication Data is available on file.

Cover design by Qualcom Design
Cover illustration: Dong Jinwen (董金文) and Danny Xuan

ISBN: 978-1-62914-777-2
Ebook ISBN: 978-1-63220-995-5
Printed in China.

Contents

The Tao of Wing Chun

Preface

Like many who are familiar with Wing Chun, my journey to the art came via Bruce Lee. Having seen Lee's films in the 1970s, millions of international fans were won over by his lithe grace and charisma, and we wanted to learn more about what he had demonstrated on the big screen. During the course of our research we learned that what Lee had practiced was his own martial creation, which he termed Jeet Kune Do, or "The Way of the Intercepting Fist." To better understand the man, we reasoned, we had better understand his art.

Unlike today, in 1973 (the year that Lee died) there wasn't anybody teaching his art. Evidently Lee had closed all three of his formal schools several years before returning to Hong Kong to focus on making the movies that would justifiably bring him international and enduring fame. Those who had assisted him in his instruction at these schools had, in an effort to both honor his memory and to preserve his art, started teaching small groups of individuals and/or teaching privately, but you had to live in either Washington or California to have access to them. As I lived in a small suburb in Ontario, Canada, such personal instruction simply wasn't going to happen. The next best thing to personal instruction from a knowledgeable teacher was self-education through studying Lee's surviving writings on his approach to martial art and its underlying philosophy, and then reinforcing his written words by re-watching his films with an eye toward more carefully examining the techniques he employed, as well as the movements and postures he made. This sustained us at the time and taught us much about

Lee's approach to martial art and, as ancillary, the Chinese martial arts in general, for many years.

Almost immediately we learned that in his youth Lee had studied a Chinese martial art called Wing Chun under the tutelage of a master by the name of Yip Man (the name would be changed to Ip Man several decades later) and one of Ip Man's senior students (and the clan's best fighter) Wong Shun Leung. When Lee wrote about Wing Chun and Ip Man he did so with great respect. In an article profiling the young martial artist in *Black Belt* magazine in 1967, Lee is quoted as saying, "I owe my achievement to my previous training in the Wing Chun style. A great style."

According to Lee's earliest students in America, such as Jesse Glover, Ed Hart, and Taky Kimura, no small portion of the principles, training methods, techniques, and philosophy that Lee employed came directly from the art of Wing Chun. That the man generally considered to be the greatest martial artist of the twentieth century should hold the art in such high regard won many of us over to it simply by default. Few of us, however, really understood the depth and breadth of the art, which was greater than we could have fathomed.

Fast forwarding to 2009, I found myself in Hong Kong working on a film about the locations that appeared in Lee's films, where I had the opportunity to meet the eldest son of Bruce Lee's teacher, the then 86-year old Ip Chun, who told me stories of his late father (who was then the subject of two feature films), the principles of the art his father taught, and how diligently the young Bruce Lee had practiced it. I resolved then that I would take up the study of the art upon my return to Canada and began immediately looking for a suitable instructor. Being older and having been involved heavily in the martial arts world at this point for thirty-some years, I had seen many—too many—fractured egos and self-professed "masters" in the various arts, and, sadly, Wing Chun seemed to me to be an art that was burdened by more than its fair share of such people. And, unfortunately for me, the nearest instruction of any substance in Wing Chun was still hundreds of miles away from where I lived. The next best thing, I reasoned, was to learn from a competent instructor on-line. After all, we were then well into the Internet age, the era of the information Super Highway, and anyone, anywhere was by some means accessible. This was how I first met Danny Xuan through his web page. Here at once was a man who downplayed his significance in the art (which was a surprising and refreshing change of pace), and yet wrote about it with such a passion and a depth of knowledge that I hadn't experienced since reading Lee's own writings on the martial way many decades earlier.

Xuan approaches his art like Lao-tzu approached nature; looking for and revealing the Tao, or underlying *way of things* in relation to human combat, much as Lao-tzu had sought to reveal it in every wave, bending branch and twinkling star. Xuan's insights were deceptively simple, which I have come to learn, is a hallmark of most truly deep subjects. He spoke of the impartial, impersonal, and yet rational natural law of things—from geometric planes to the nature of force production—to which all things abide in accordance with their true selves or natural natures. From the perspective of the Tao, all of the laws of nature are united and their aggregate is simply reality, in which all natural forces, forms, and structures find their proper place and optimal method of operating and surviving. Apparent contradictions and diversities seem to dissolve before it. It is a means by which one learns to understand, trust, and act in accordance with ways of nature.

> There is nothing weaker than water
> But none is superior to it in overcoming the hard,
> For which there is no substitute.
> That weakness overcomes strength
> And gentleness overcomes rigidity,
> No one does not know;
> No one can put into practice. [1]

Although these words sound as though they were written by Bruce Lee (most certainly he adopted them as the cornerstone of his martial philosophy), tradition has it that they were first written by Lao-tzu in the fifth century BCE. And while they do reveal a truth about human combat, they also reveal a larger truth about the reality of the world and how its various elements interact.

Xuan understands this bigger picture and his interpretation of the art of Wing Chun is a product of this understanding. Coming from a traditional background where he was simply taught the methods and postures of the art, he wasn't satisfied and instead of merely continuing on practicing by rote, he retired from running a very successful business on the West Coast of Canada to backpack his way across China. Along the way he would stop in small villages that tourists never see and that are seldom if ever written about, and look more deeply into the culture that had produced his art. But more importantly, he began thinking about his art in a different way, examining every aspect of it—from its legendary origin, to its fundamental stances, to its forms, to its conceptual underpinnings. At the end of his trek he was a different man with a different and more profound understanding of the art of Wing Chun. It is this understanding that he shares with the reader in this book. In an attempt to get at the actual "Tao" of the art, he examines the natural laws regarding structure and forces. Indeed, the chapter on forces (Chapter Eleven) may well contain the distilled essence of Wing Chun, for as Xuan once told me, "This art is also about life. And life is about dealing with forces. And in our lives we're always dealing with some kind of force or some kind of conflict, whether it be with, you know, your wife, your brothers, sisters, or your boss in business, there's always some kind of challenges that you're going to have to face." This is perhaps the most technical chapter in the book and, to some, perhaps, intimidating, but like Lao-tzu's book, it repays further reading and re-reading.

Unlike other books on Wing Chun that have appeared over the years, and that for the most part provide but a surface examination of the art, Xuan takes the reader as deep into the art as the reader may wish to go, revealing its many components and the interrelatedness (in true Yin-Yang fashion) of its concepts. With the greatest respect for the founders of the art, Xuan presents the reasons (heretofore absent from print) why the art came into being, the nature of its methods, and the natural sciences that underpin every facet of the Wing Chun system. To the seasoned student of Wing Chun, his insights will represent a breath of fresh air and a welcome voice in what had previously become a musty corridor of echoes from the past.

While I am listed as the co-author of this title it should be clarified that the ideas and content revealed in this book is not the result of a collaboration between two people; the content herein represents Danny Xuan's singular achievement. My contribution, if you'd care to call it that, has been in the form of how the material has been presented—not its substance.

The Tao of Wing Chun in my opinion reveals the results of one man's dedicated search for the real truth that underpins his art. And, if I may have the audacity to amend the words of Lao-tzu, here, at least, is one man who can "put into practice" the principles expressed through that Tao. It has taken him over forty years to accomplish this, and another two years to distill it down to its essence and communicate it to you within these pages. Hopefully this book will allow the reader to learn more about the art of Wing Chun, and, more importantly, to learn more about yourself, than you might have been previously aware.

—John Little

INTRODUCTION

O VER THE DECADES THERE have been plenty of books written about the Chinese martial art of Wing Chun, so what more could possibly be said about it? Plenty!

Most Wing Chun books follow a certain theme, style, and pattern that the first books on Karate started in the late nineteen fifties and early sixties, such as Masutatsu Oyama's *What is Karate?* and *This is Karate!* or Masatoshi Nakayam's *Dynamic Karate*. Before these books, there were some Chinese language martial arts books that focused on the shadow boxing forms of the various arts, but they discussed almost no applicable techniques. There were also some English language books written on the arts of Jujitsu and Judo, but they focused solely on the techniques and applications of these arts, owing to the fact that there were no forms or katas within their respective systems. Those first Karate books were both comprehensive and complete; they covered the fundamental principles of the art, its stances and postures, as well as which body parts were to be used for striking, and which of your opponent's body parts served as the best targets to strike. They were essentially catalogues of striking (offensive) and blocking (defensive) techniques, counter-attack (defensive and offensive) techniques, as well as applicable techniques for street confrontations, such as what to do against multiple assailants. These books also included stretching exercises, strength-building exercises, bag- or pad-striking exercises and movements from the katas (or forms) of their art.

The first comprehensive book on Wing Chun that came after some small introductory books in the late sixties and early seventies was Leung Ting's *Wing Tsun Kuen*, which was published in 1978. It followed the big

Karate-book format revealing the forms, techniques, and applications of Wing Chun. Although other big and comprehensive books followed, they conformed to the same format and in any case merely touched upon the surface of the art of Wing Chun. They were heavy on photos, but short on text; dense with techniques, but short on their conceptual underpinnings.

In this book, I wish to delve into the inner depths of my art of Wing Chun, and present the crucially important principles that photo books by their very nature must leave out.

And this lack of presenting the underlying principles of a martial art is not simply a defect found in books. Indeed, one of the faults that I find prevalent in most martial arts schools is that they don't teach their students the principles of their systems. A new student is typically thrown into a class and told to follow the teacher's (or lead student's) movements. The student learns drill after drill, and techniques are taught to them later, but with little explanation. Students are never given an opportunity to question the drills or the techniques they are being made to perform. A new student is naturally inquisitive, and will have many questions in his mind, but when he is not given the opportunity to vocalize these queries he soon loses his curiosity and becomes an automaton.

Why are these principles not taught? In many cases, it is because the system does not have any. Many of these arts offer the prospective student an impressive artifice that is built upon some very fragmented ideas with an even more fragmented foundation. This is especially true of the more recent hybrid "arts" created by people who think largely about accumulating techniques from various styles rather than looking for root truths of human movement in combat. In other cases, the teacher may simply be unaware of the principles of his art. These teachers may have studied their martial art blindly over the decades, coming to understand only its superficial move-ments. And then there is the commercialism that comes into play in most martial arts. In order to make money from teaching or instructing, one must have a lot of students. However, if an instructor is able to achieve this, he is then in a position where he is unable to provide individual attention to his students. In order to grow enrollment and sustain a large member-ship, a special system must then be put in place to teach a large group and to keep them interested and coming in for instruction.

The belt (ranking) system that is in play in most martial arts, although originally intended for grading and goal setting, is nowadays often used as bait to keep students hooked as ongoing paying customers. Training a large group class tends to offer the student very little in terms of content (in the martial arts sense), as one spends most of one's time warming up, stretching and building muscle, which you could actually do elsewhere at aerobic classes or strength-training gymnasiums. In the new martial arts studios one typically will spend the first twenty minutes warming up, and then spend another twenty minutes on drills, another twenty minutes on kata or forms, and then, perhaps, fifteen minutes may be devoted to technique training. Finally, sparring might be done, but if it is, only for about ten minutes or so. At the very end of the class, perhaps five minutes might be devoted to what they term "cool-down" exercises. There's nothing wrong with this approach—if your goal in taking up a martial art is simply to exercise your body and do a little martial arts on the side. However, if you are serious about learning martial arts, shouldn't you be spending more time on it in class? If you want to learn to golf, you would expect your instructor to teach you golfing, not aerobics, calisthenics, or gymnastics. What would you say to him if he were to tell you that you would be doing an hour and fifteen minutes of calisthenics but only fifteen minutes of golf instruction? A proper martial arts class (and particularly a proper Wing Chun class) should be focused instead on the practical application of combat techniques and concepts. You should do fitness exercises on your own; there is no sense in spending your time doing them in Wing Chun class. As for the drills, there are some in Wing Chun, but they are not the same type that other martial arts systems teach. Wing Chun drills are performed with a partner to develop sensitivity, reflex action, and to sharpen one's combative techniques. Most schools make students drill on blocks, punches, and stances that are simply impractical, ineffective, and unrealistic. The students in such schools will quickly discover that they are unable to use any of what they have been practicing even in their sparring, let alone in a real life-or-death situation. The contorted postures, the low stances, the hard blocks, and the weird-shaped hand strikes are totally useless. Yet, schools continue teaching these things, and students continue practicing them.

Most drills in most martial arts styles consist of "pattern" training, known as "kata" in Japanese, and "heung" in Korean. Patterns were originally created for martial arts students to practice the techniques of their art without a partner. They are only beneficial if the moves that are being practiced are actually applicable in sparring or real fighting. If not, they are a waste of time. This is true with most martial arts patterns. In fact, in the Japanese arts such as karate, students will learn about ten sets of patterns before acquiring their black belt. Once they obtain their black belt they will learn even more. More complex moves are then added to their growing repertoire—and most of these are useless in a real fight situation. Don't get me wrong; there is nothing wrong with patterns if they are training you to perform practical techniques, but they are a waste of time, effort, and energy if they contain nothing but impractical movements.

In the Wing Chun system, as passed on from Great-Grandmaster Ip Man's lineage, there are six forms in total; three open-hand forms, one training apparatus form, and two weapons forms. All of the movements in each of these forms are functional and can be used practically. In addition, they will train the practitioner in becoming a holistic martial artist.

THE FORMS WITHIN WING CHUN

The first form is an open-hand form called Siu Nim Tau (小念頭), literally the "Little Study Head," or "the beginning of one's studies," the first lessons or fundamental teachings. The second form is called "Chum Kiu" (尋橋), or "Seeking the Bridge," and reflects the intermediate path that the practitioner needs to enter before bridging on to the advanced level of "Biu Jee" (鏢指) or "Hurling Fingers." In Siu Nim Tau, the practitioner learns to solidify his structure and ground himself firmly. The movements train him to isolate and coordinate different parts of his arm in a relaxed, flowing and sensitive manner. This form introduces the practitioner to the principles of Wing Chun, the defensive and offensive arsenals of the system, and provides instructions on how to use these arsenals, and also provides the student with examples of their usage. In the Siu Nim Tau training level, there are drills and exercises that go with the form that allow the practitioner to manifest the knowledge acquired from the form into hands-on practicality. The knowledge acquired from the drills and exercises is then applied and tested through sparring. In terms of warfare, the Siu Nim Tau–level practitioners are the foot soldiers that are trained to guard and destroy opponents attacking one's "fort" or body. Continuing on with our metaphor, the Chum Kiu–level practitioners are the cavaliers that fight and tread over enemies in the battlefield, while the Biu Jee–level practitioners are the Special Forces that penetrate forts, and seek out and destroy the commander of the opposing force.

When a practitioner completes the three open-hand forms, he moves onto the Muk Yan Jong (木人樁) level, or the wooden man (or wooden dummy) apparatus form. Here, he will be trained to become a bombardier. He will break through all barriers and learn how to completely destroy his enemy's forts.

The two weapon forms that follow were designed not so much for weapon fighting as for adding elements that mold the practitioner into fulfilling his ultimate potential as a martial artist. The original creators of the Wing Chun system understood that all weapons ultimately become obsolete. For example, what chance does a nine-foot pole or a pair of arm-length knives have against guns these days? For that matter, what chance did they have against spears, arrows, or poisonous darts in the old days? The 6.5 Pole form was designed not for pole fighting but rather to develop supreme punching power in the practitioner. When a practitioner has that, he will eliminate his opponent within seconds—just like Mike Tyson did in his prime. The Twin Swords or Knives form contains information that reveals everything a practitioner needs to know about Wing Chun, but in a condensed form. In terms of warfare, the practitioner of the 6.5 Pole belongs to the artillery force, and the sword-form "Bat Jum Do" (八斬刀)—"Eight Severing Sword"—practitioner is the ultimate assassin; he is discreet, moves invisibly and penetrates into the chambers of the king without detection. He severs the king's head, and, by so doing, singly defeats the whole nation.

One thing must be said though; Wing Chun is not all about warfare. Wing Chun offers many things to many people because of its holistic approach. For some, it offers a course on ancient Chinese art and culture, such as the philosophies of Confucius, Laozi (author of the *Tao Te Ch'ing*), Sun Tzu (author of *The Art of War*), and Traditional Chinese Medicine. For others, it provides a means to acquire self-defense skills, flexibility, coordination, stamina, as well as enhancing one's physical and mental fitness. In addition, it helps the practitioner develop humility, focus, determination, self-discipline, self-esteem, self-respect, confidence, character, camaraderie, and a means to access our untapped strengths. Foremost, it offers the practitioner the ability to apply Wing Chun principles to daily life. After all, isn't life about dealing with physical and mental challenges?

—Danny Xuan

ONE

WING CHUN: A REALITY CHECK

WING CHUN IS UNIQUE among all other martial arts and, owing to this uniqueness, it is not surprising to discover that it is an art that is widely misunderstood. In comparison to most other martial arts, Wing Chun arrived quite late onto the scene, long after other arts had been exposed to the public (especially in the West). Consequently, the public, commentators in the martial arts media and practitioners of other arts looked upon Wing Chun through the filters of their own preconceptions of what a martial art should be. When some of these people decided to take up the study of Wing Chun, they typically brought along all of their previous conceptions and experiences, and expected to practice Wing Chun as they would any of the other arts they had studied in the past, which, unfortunately, is not the best way to understand Wing Chun's concepts, principles, and training methods.

What is it about Wing Chun that makes it unique in martial arts, and why do most practitioners generally miss the boat when it comes to understanding and perfecting this art? While there are many answers to these questions, to even understand these questions, the individual seeking to thoroughly understand Wing Chun must understand the full implications of the following points:

- It is the only martial art in all of martial arts history that was created by women, and/or was developed from a woman's perspective. Men

[1]

often reject the female aspect of the art, and approach it solely from a man's point of view.

- The (shadow boxing) forms of Wing Chun were designed to deceive laymen and other martial artists. In other words, what you see is definitely *not* what you get. The forms are actually Wing Chun's secret "user manuals," with hidden messages of the system encrypted within them. Practitioners of other arts who watch the Wing Chun forms always tend to interpret the forms superficially and then rationalize away the movements with the most obvious explanations. The founders of the Wing Chun system accomplished exactly what they had intended; to keep the art a secret, and to fool those who didn't fit the Wing Chun family profile.
- Unlike most other martial arts that train practitioners to read an opponent's intent and action using only their sense of vision, and then automate a certain reaction against a certain type of attack, Wing Chun trains its practitioners to read an opponent's action through tactile sense, and to react intuitively and intelligently against any action or change within a given combative situation.

With these essential points now presented, let's move on to consider for a moment what Wing Chun *is not*.

- It is not what's presented and perceived in any of the Wing Chun movies made to date
- It is not what's presented and perceived in the popular Ip Man movies
- It is not what's presented and perceived in television programs
- It is not what's typically presented and perceived in YouTube videos
- It is not what is presented in most books on Wing Chun
- It is not flamboyant or spectacular
- It is not a fighting style
- It is not calisthenics
- It is not acrobatics
- It is not a sport

And while I'm at it, this is as good a time as any to correct a few more misconceptions:

- Wing Chun does not empower you to become invincible against twenty, ten, or even a single opponent (in reality, no martial art can do this)
- You will not magically inherit the skills of a grandmaster by touching hands with him, hanging out with him, adopting his habits, or being associated with him

- You will not necessarily become skillful even if you've trained under the best sifu (teacher) in the world
- And here's the capper: A grandmaster is not necessarily grand in skill or knowledge

I'm fully convinced that if my late Great-Grandmaster Ip Man rose up from the dead, he'd laugh himself to death seeing what the movies have made him out to be—and then he'd dive right back into his coffin after seeing how Wing Chun is now being represented, corrupted, diluted, and practiced. And while this is only my opinion, I believe that he would be somewhat embarrassed to face his Wing Chun forefathers who would likely scold him for opening the art of Wing Chun to the masses, and allowing the art to get bastardized and poisoned to such a state of present disarray.

It must be remembered that movies and television programs are made primarily for entertainment purposes by conglomerates and tycoons for the sole purpose of generating megadollars, rather than to advance facts, truth, or reality. Their purpose, of course, is to twist and fictionalize reality, create illusions and stimulate human emotion by transporting the viewing audience away from reality. Such films and television programs are made to entertain people, which is fine, however when they present a martial art such as Wing Chun, the viewer must keep in mind that what he or she is seeing has been sensationalized for entertainment purposes. Quite simply, the martial art action sequences in these various media presentations do not reflect the true principles of the art. The Wing Chun system prides itself in being economical, efficient, and direct. It does this by training the practitioner to use all of his limbs simultaneously to defend and attack. In Wing Chun, defense and attack is one synchronized unit—not two separate entities. In the movies, there are far too many blocks and strikes executed, and even these are performed inefficiently, unproductively, and indicate the use of too much energy. Where is the efficiency and productivity when the lead character throws a dozen punches to the opponent's chest—and still leaves him standing to fight back? Where is the economy of motion, the efficiency and productivity, when the lead character requires ten full minutes to eliminate his opponent? When one knocks out or immobilizes a person within three moves in as many seconds, then one is demonstrating simplicity, directness, and efficiency in fighting. Even if it took you ten movements to finish off an opponent in thirty seconds, you're still far better off than executing three hundred movements in three minutes. If you find yourself pitted against an opponent who is bigger and stronger than you, or up against more than one opponent, you have a very small window of opportunity to walk out of the fight successfully (or to walk out at all). The longer you spend exchanging

[3]

blows, missing opportunities, and wasting your energy, the more opportunities you will present to your opponent(s) to defeat you. Consequently, a Wing Chun practitioner must learn to move economically and efficiently, and to be able to hit powerfully at an opponent's vital points in order to successfully immobilize, maim, or kill that opponent within a handful of movements and a matter of seconds.

Most of the documentaries on Wing Chun are typically researched, written, and directed by non-Wing Chun practitioners. They are typically enamored by the mystic and spectacular-looking movements of the martial arts, and present their documentaries that way. They feature and interview the best-known Wing Chun personalities—not necessarily the best Wing Chun practitioners. The best Wing Chun people that I've encountered over the years are usually low-key, while the best-known are those with spectacular marketing skills rather than spectacular Kung Fu skills. They make Wing Chun appear spectacular visually, when, in reality, it is not a flashy art. For a system to be economical, efficient, and productive, its techniques must appear to be very minimalistic—because they are. In all the years that my Great-Grandmaster Ip Man practiced and taught Wing Chun, and with all the skills he possessed, he never once demonstrated Wing Chun publicly in the movies, television, or books. I believe that in his later years he consented to one magazine interview, and was mentioned in some of the Hong Kong newspapers. In his final weeks, he succumbed to being photographed and filmed under the condition that the film and images would not be published nor distributed to the general public (with the perhaps predictable result that these photographs and films are now readily available over the Internet).

Today, you will find ample documentaries, advertisements, and instructional videos on Wing Chun. With the advent of YouTube, you can find hundreds of video clips showing practitioners teaching and demonstrating Wing Chun, most of them with very little knowledge and training, but presenting themselves for their minute of worldwide exposure. One of their most common demonstrations is the "one-inch punch" made famous by the late Bruce Lee. Unbeknownst to them, the one-inch punch is not a product of Wing Chun (although the concept underlying it is very compatible with Wing Chun principles) but rather was a technique that was unique to Bruce Lee's personal Kung Fu exhibitions.

Wing Chun teaches the practitioner to throw a punch from whatever position the fist is at without cocking the arm back. The fist can be one yard, one foot, or one inch away from the opponent. The power in Wing Chun punching is generated from the practitioner's waist and pelvis, which is sent down to the ground and then bounced back up to propel the arm and fist forward. Bruce Lee demonstrated this principle in public, adding some drama to it by placing a chair behind the recipient of his punch so that the recipient would be driven backwards and fall over it. Now, almost every one-inch-punch demo includes the chair gimmick. I've even seen some real creative presentations that have the recipient of the punch being knocked through a plywood plank that is being held by spotters. I grant you that this looks spectacular to those who don't know any better, but the truth of the matter is that when a punch sends a person several steps backwards, it's actually just a strong push, not a punch. The force of the thrust simply propels its recipient backwards through the air instead of delivering it through his body and into the ground. It's the same difference as striking a golf ball through the air with a baseball bat, versus smashing it down into the ground. With all the boxing knockouts you've seen, I bet you haven't seen any that made the guy stagger back 5 steps and fall down cold. A real knockout punch hardly moves the guy back at all; it usually drops the guy right on the spot, or at most, he may take one step back before falling. So, the one-inch punch that flings the guy back several steps does just that—it *flings* him, but it certainly doesn't hurt him. One YouTube "one-inch-punch" demo by a well-known Wing Chun teacher shows him winding his fist back at least 12-inches (not one-inch) to break a one-inch pinewood board (the same boards that seven-year-olds learn to break in Taekwondo demonstrations). I've looked at that video several times, slowing it down to confirm the distance his arm travels. It is so obvious that I can't imagine anyone being fooled by it.

And then there is the unfortunately all-too-common demo that shows a "master" pounding the crap out of one of his students who is made to throw just one lame punch or kick, which is usually initiated from well outside of the proper range for throwing such a technique. The student throws his one punch and then freezes on the spot, while his master responds with five or six counterattacks, finishing him off by taking him down to the floor and then slapping the student with another five or six shots. These "masters" are in denial! They imagine themselves as movie stars, and perform this demo so often that they begin to believe in their own pretentious prowess. If any of these actors ever got into a real fight in the street, he would have a very rude awakening; his opponents would no longer be attacking him from outside of harm's range or take falls for him—and the fights would no longer be choreographed for him to win. In real life, your opponent will be relentlessly aggressive, with the full intent to hurt or kill you. Faced with such an opponent, such a "master" would suddenly discover that the techniques he had used on his less-aggressive helpers would no longer be effective. His punches would not hurt his opponent, but his opponent's punches would definitely hurt him. Those who are in denial will be even more unprepared and shocked than those who have never fought before and who don't fantasize about themselves as supermen.

While the art of Karate has a distinctive history because of its relatively young age and clear records, Wing Chun's history is shrouded in mystery both because of its older age and because of the general secrecy that attended its arrival into the martial arts world. Although there are vague verbal histories on Wing Chun, they cannot be verified and positively confirmed as facts. So, if one wants to write about Wing Chun's past, one must clearly state that it is based on a story that has been passed down orally over the centuries. Unfortunately, most Wing Chun stories are hearsay, but often presented as if they were facts.

Apart from the Wing Chun's vague history, compared to Karate's clear-cut history, its forms are also unclear compared to Karate's straightforward forms. Karate forms (kata) are exercises designed to drill the practitioners in the stances, blocks and strikes that make up Karate techniques. There are many types of Karate, and each type might have upwards of twenty to thirty katas. Overall, they are movements for defense and attack that are performed as if one was fighting against one or more imaginary opponents. They are straightforward: What you see is what you get.

The Wing Chun from Great-Grandmaster Ip Man's lineage has but six forms in total. However, these six forms have much more behind them than just fighting techniques. Indeed, the Wing Chun forms have nothing to do with fighting imaginary opponents. In fact, the Wing Chun forms were designed to fool people who spied on the art into thinking that it was a very lame fighting art. In other words, what you see is *not* what you get. The founders of Wing Chun encrypted many hidden messages in the movements of the forms that are unknown to even the most ardent of Wing Chun practitioners. Although these practitioners have produced books and videos showing how a particular Wing Chun form is to be performed, it prevents any clear explanation for the movements they are performing. At best, they explain the movements of the forms as fighting applications in the most obvious and simplistic what-you-see-is-what-you-get manner by placing a person in front, behind, or at the side of a movement from the form, and calling the movement performed a strike, block or kick. Even a child could come up with such explanations! If the founders of Wing Chun wished the art to be secretive, they certainly wouldn't have designed the forms to be deciphered so easily. Those of us who've practiced Wing Chun for many decades know how clever the founders were in developing such an ingenious system. Such inspired masters must also have had the ingenuity to encrypt it.

So, if Wing Chun is not a fighting style, and if the form movements are not application based, then what is Wing Chun and what are the purposes of the movements in its forms? To understand this, you must first understand how the martial arts first began.

TWO

Genesis: The Origin of Martial Art

U NLESS A MARTIAL ART was created in the last hundred years (such as Aikido, Judo, Karate, Taekwondo, and Jeet Kune Do), its origin will be hard to trace with any degree of exactitude. Consequently, the origins of older martial arts such as Shaolin, Chen Tai Chi, Bagua, and Wing Chun are shrouded in mystery.

Some historians believe that the martial art practiced at the Shaolin Temple in China was actually created by an Indian Buddhist monk called Bodidharma, but others do not. It is not clear when the art of Tai Chi was created or by whom exactly, but we do know that it was brought to prominence in the Chen Village by a person named Chen Wanting in the seventeenth century. Bagua's origin is also unclear: Dong Haichuan, the first known practitioner of the art, claimed to have learned it from a mysterious master. Wing Chun is thought to have been formulated by an abbess named Ng Mui, who taught Yim Wing Chun, who went on to develop it further with her husband Leung Bokchao. In each of the above cases, the stories of the respective art's origins were initially passed down via an oral tradition and then eventually they were committed to writing.

Whenever the origins of something are unclear, people feel uncomfortable with such vagueness and like to speculate about how such things as fire or simple machines originated. Typically, such things begin accidentally (or incidentally) and are only understood initially by the brightest minds of the

[9]

time, who then utilize these discoveries to the benefit of either themselves or their societies. As societies grow or change, variations are required and, out of this, the original discoveries are then modified to keep pace with the present need. This type of evolution occurs across all fields, from science and art, to philosophy, politics, and commerce. There were no "schools" for any of these fields in the beginning; the schools always came later.

In my humble opinion, it only stands to reason that the martial arts evolved in a similar manner. No super being or manual fell from the sky to start a martial arts school. It seems more plausible that someone from a small community may have gotten into more fights than others did in his community, and this individual ended up winning his fights more often than losing them. The more he fought, the more experience he gained, and the more fights he won, the more renowned he became. And the more renowned he became, the more challenges he received. Eventually, when he grew old and his testosterone levels had waned, he became less aggressive and combative. He began to fight less and even to refuse challenges. Although he was famous in his youth, young fighters were no longer interested in challenging him because there was no longer anything to be gained by such an encounter. If they were to fight with him and win, people would mock them for bullying an old man. If they were to fight with him and lose, people would mock them for losing to an old man. However, the old fighter still had his reputation, a reputation based upon decades of successful fighting experience. He was looked upon by members of the community as a man who may have some tips and secrets that he employed to help him win his encounters, and that he might be willing to share. The young men recognize now that there is more to be gained by learning from him than by fighting him. And so the old man is approached by one or more of these people and asked to share his knowledge of fighting with them.

As far as the old fighter is concerned, he has nothing to teach; he had fought each and every opponent according to their abilities and size, the environment and circumstances also played a role, as did the issue of what weapons were available to him. He may have first refused the notion of teaching students, however, after pondering the idea, he decided to teach them more to pacify his own curiosity than theirs. While the students were interested in learning his fighting methodology, he was more interested in coming to understand just how he had overcome the various opponents he had encountered throughout his life. Perhaps he began by analyzing all of his fights and examining the various strikes he used and when and how he used them. From there he might have examined the possible reasons why he won some fights and lost others. After reflecting on this for some time, he might believe that he has pinpointed a common denominator in the fights that he won, and a thought begins to form in his mind of the concept of fighting itself and of what actions and approaches typically resulted in a win, and what actions and approaches typically resulted in a loss.

However, just sharing these concepts with his students wasn't going to be enough. They wouldn't be able to defend themselves equipped with just a concept or two—they needed experience. However, sending them out to fight would not be proper or productive. He decided that he had to devise a training program that would not only manifest his concepts, but also provide his students with practical experience that would better prepare them for the reality of fighting. And along with the insights that he had gleaned from his fighting experiences over the years, he also wanted to impart the virtues he had gained as both a fighter and a human being.

Although the martial art master was possessed of much wisdom and experience, he had to find a way to pass this on to his students in a much shorter period of time than it had taken him to acquire. So, he may have first designed a course of sorts that would communicate to his students the principles of his fighting concept. The course would have introduced the students to the principles and tools required to implement his concept. Then he might have shown them how to apply these principles and concepts by providing his students with an array of exercises in order to help develop their skills, and, finally, a means by which they could apply this knowledge in a real fight situation.

As with most students, some probably grasped his concept of fighting very well, while others did not. Some may have become skilled fighters, while others did not (whether they grasped his concept or not). Similarly, not everyone who grasped his concept or became good fighters became good teachers. Every student turned out differently under the same master. Eventually, when the master died, some of his students might have opted to teach others. And they, in turn, produced students who were different again. From one generation to the next, certain students turned out to be exceptional, while others only mediocre. Some went on to revise the original concept and training program of the master, while others spun off to create an entirely new concept altogether.

Meanwhile, in villages elsewhere the same evolution was taking place; however, the fighters-turned-masters all had different concepts of fighting based upon their different life experiences. They, in turn, produced students possessed of different fighting concepts and training programs.

When their small communities became villages, and the villages became a kingdom, the ruler sought to employ the more skilled fighters as bodyguards and trainers for the kingdom's army. However, these fighters had never taught large groups before, and so they struggled with the teaching program that they had used so successfully with smaller groups. Consequently, they redesigned the training program to suit the army, thus transforming an individualistic civilian art into a martial art. The individualist art was preserved for the royal family members and high-ranking officials while the new filtered art was regimented to the soldiers. It became even more filtered as it was passed down to the lower echelons. In order to maintain control and order over the citizens, the fighting arts became exclusive to the government. Civilians were banned from practicing them.

Each family, village, or kingdom had its own unique martial art system. To improve their systems, the various martial arts schools spied upon each other. They planted spies, bribed, and wooed students from one school to defect to another. To prevent the secrets from leaking out, new security methods were then devised. Written documents were discarded since they could be damaged, stolen, or replicated. Clever masters then designed shadowboxing forms for their students to practice, but these forms had messages encrypted in the movements, which were only known to the most trusted students. The forms were designed to deceive the spies, almost to the point of being the exact opposite of what they appeared to be, with the result that only the most experienced and cleverest martial artists could crack the code and decipher them. To be certain, not all masters thought of encrypting their forms. Most of them created the what-you-see-is-what-you-get type. Nevertheless, it was important that even these should be hidden away from the spying eyes of competing schools and practitioners of other arts.

During the warring periods one kingdom conquered another. The officers of the conquered kingdom often became insurgents; training civilians to become fighters. As a result, the laymen, who were banned from practicing martial arts and carrying weapons, began to develop their own fighting arts using both household and farming tools. Thus, the real unadulterated fighting arts came full circle back to their original practitioners: the civilians.

When more peaceful periods returned, there were cultural exchanges between one kingdom and another, and the secrecy of the arts became lax, with martial artists now teaching and practicing their respective arts more openly. Many did it simply for exercise and appreciation for the art, while a few took it more seriously and with one eye trained toward commerce. Among those who took up study of the arts, some became modestly skilled, and a few became superbly skilled. However, with the arrival of sophisticated long-range weapons, martial artists were now no longer considered to be as valuable or respectable to have around. Royal bodyguards and masters began losing their jobs. If they were fortunate, the best of these martial artists sought and found employment from wealthy merchants who hired them on as bodyguards and teachers. The rest of them made a humble living teaching small groups, or became performers on the stage or in the streets. This group consisted of very good to very poor martial artists.

This, I believe, is how the various martial arts have come down to us today. There are so many different kinds of martial arts that are now exposed to us via globalization and the Internet. And there are millions of martial arts practitioners, but very, very few of these practitioners are knowledgeable, fewer still are good at teaching, and fewest of all are those who are skilled in fighting. A martial artist that embodies all three of these characteristics is exceptionally rare.

OLD WINE IN NEW SKINS

The richest period of martial arts, which I would refer to as being the martial arts renaissance, took place in China during the latter period of the Ming Dynasty (sixteenth century) to the middle part of the Qing Dynasty (eighteenth century). These were the Warring and Revolutionary Periods, and during these periods probably all humanly possible defensive and offensive techniques were tested and brought to the highest level.

The best and best-known fighters were challenged regularly in those times. These fights were not like today's rule-based competitions where you can end a fight by tapping out and walk away unhurt with lots of money in your pocket. These ancient fights included a death-liability waiver, or, at the very least, the surrender of a school and its students to the winner. I'd wager that few if any of today's MMA competitors would believe themselves skilled enough to go into a no-rules and no-money competition that included a death-liability waiver. The ancient fighters, with such high stakes, thought it necessary to prepare themselves against a variety of fighting styles. Today's martial artists haven't come up with anything new by mixing various arts together. The truth of the matter is that the ancient fighters were already mixing various martial arts. They had to in order to fight martial artists from different systems. Some brought in as many techniques as they could from other systems into their own, while others took in only those that adhered to the principles of their system.

Many of today's top MMA fighters come from traditional martial arts schools, and attribute their success to the training, experience and discipline from their respective arts. Anderson Silva was a black-belt Taekwondo practitioner before entering into cage fights. *Black Belt* Magazine's 2009 Fighter of the Year, Lyoto Machida, is a Shotokan Karate practitioner. Ronda Rousey's background is in Judo. She was the Bronze medalist in the 2008 Olympics. The Gracie family, which dominated the UFC and Octagon platforms in the early years of their conceptions, adhered strictly to Brazilian Jujitsu. George

St. Pierre trained in Kyokushin Karate, and wore a third-degree black belt. In an April 24, 2013, *SB Nation* article, he is quoted as saying in an interview with Joe Rogan that, "It has nothing to do with wrestling. How I get in and out is because of my Karate. People are like, 'no way, Karate, no.' And I'm like, 'yes.' Karate allows me to cut the distance and take the people down. It's because of my leg, the way I do it, and the timing is because of my Karate. I wrestle too, but my karate is primary." The person who thinks that he can just go into any MMA school, learn some techniques, and walk into the ring or the cage for a match, is likely go home with a concussion instead of a gold belt and the bullion he had expected. So don't think for a moment that we're living in a martial arts renaissance period presently just because we have thousands of schools and millions of practitioners, or because Hollywood, Hong Kong, and Cable TV are producing a multitude of shows featuring martial arts and martial artists. In fact, this is more an indication that martial art, per se, is now at its nadir rather than its zenith. When every Tom, Dick, and Harry is now a sensei, sifu, grandmaster, or great-grandmaster, you know that the martial arts are not experiencing the richest period of quality in their history.

I believe that authentic martial art pretty much died out in the nineteenth century. With the introduction of Western imperialism and guns into China, close-range weapons and hand-to-hand-combat arts were bound to fade into oblivion. The best of the martial artists at the time were no match against guns. Slowly but surely the martial arts began to decline in China. Those who relied on them professionally were reduced to the level of street or stage performers. And the generations that followed simply produced more performers—not fighters.

Having said this, there were some masters during these periods that continued to value and preserve their respective arts, with the result that their arts are still alive today. Through the years, some masters modified their arts, while others attempted to maintain the original art as it was first taught to them. And this is not to suggest that any one art is necessarily any better than any other. However, as with all things, there are systems that work better than others. For example, although all automobiles operate under the umbrella of mechanical technology, manufacturers have built them differently in order to suit different needs. Some vehicles are built for better fuel economy, others for greater speed, comfort, durability, aesthetics, or lower cost. However, within each classification there has always been one manufacturer that produced a better product than the others because of superior design and execution. And superior design comes from a better understanding and application of the physical laws and mechanical science that underpins automobile construction. Some manufacturers have even accomplished the designing of cars that are fast, comfortable, durable, aesthetically pleasing, and economical—all at the same time.

Similarly, martial arts were designed under the umbrella of physical science and biomechanics. The creators of these arts may have originally designed them for physical health, mental health, spiritual health, longevity, sexual prowess, character building, self-defense, external strength, internal strength, close-range fighting, long-range fighting, ground fighting, short-term usage, and long-term usage. And within these various classifications, some systems excelled far beyond the others. However, like the car with all the qualities I indicated, a single martial art system may likewise contain the means to successfully develop all of the objectives indicated above. Such a system of martial art would be considered holistic.

It is my personal opinion that Wing Chun is just such an art; it is in my opinion one of the best, one of the most holistic and one of the most practical martial arts ever created. Now before anyone starts knocking on my door to challenge me, I'll restate my belief that Wing Chun is ONE of the best, one of the most holistic, and one of the most practical martial arts ever created. Sad to say, but most other martial arts are not as holistic and nowhere near as practical. Why? To answer that question, we first have to understand the evolution of modern martial arts.

THREE

MARTIAL ART: THE CHINESE CONNECTION

MOST MARTIAL ARTS HISTORIANS will not dispute that martial arts developed to the richest and highest level in China between the seventeenth and nineteenth centuries. Historically, China and Japan have always had a love/hate relationship with each other; they have warred against each other at times and exchanged cultures at other times. Even during the peaceful periods, they were suspicious of each other. Today, it remains the same.

China had enjoyed a good relationship with its neighbor, the Ryukyu Kingdom. The Ryukyu Kingdom was a tribute state of China, meaning that it paid China tribute (tax or protection money, so to speak), as was customary such as Rome's relationship to its vassal states. In fact, the relationship between China and the Ryukyu Kingdom was so good that many Chinese migrated to the Ryukyu Kingdom and the two countries traded and exchanged cultures. Part of this cultural exchange was the introduction into the Ryukyu Kingdom of Chinese martial arts. At that time the Chinese martial arts were simply called Kara Te (唐手), meaning "Chinese Hand (fighting)." The character 唐, pronounced *Kara* in Japanese, is pronounced *Tang* in Chinese and was the moniker for the Chinese during the Tang Dynasty era.

In 1879, Japan annexed the Ryukyu Kingdom and renamed it Okinawa (as it is known today). And by the turn of the twentieth century there were many Okinawan Kara Te practitioners. In 1922 one of the practitioners, Gichin Funakoshi, was invited to Tokyo by the Japanese ministry of education to give them a demonstration with the intent of implementing Kara Te into the Japanese university curriculum. Within a few years, all major universities in Tokyo had Kara Te programs.

In 1935, Gichin Funakoshi and a group of Kara Te practitioners formed the Japan Karate Association, and opened the first official Kara Te school (or dojo) in Tokyo, called Shotokan. Because of the Japanese patriotic fervor and military expansion at the time, Funakoshi changed the character that meant "Chinese," Kara (唐), with another character sounding the same, Kara (空), meaning "empty," thus changing the name of the art to "Empty Hand (Fighting)." He also changed the names of the forms (kata) to break the association with the original Chinese.

Japanese Judo, Jujitsu, Kendo, Aikido and other arts were all spinoffs from the introduction of the Chinese martial arts through Okinawa, just as Taekwondo is a spinoff from Karate. From 1910 to 1945 Japan occupied Korea and that was how Karate was introduced into Korea. Moreover, many Koreans were sent to Tokyo for education, where they learned Karate. Although Korea had its own local fighting arts, mainly consisting of kicks (the roots of which all stemmed from China as well), Taekwondo was formulated in 1955 under the leadership of General Choi Hong Hi, who had been trained in Karate.

One of the points to consider as we examine the history of modern martial arts is how much information the Chinese actually divulged to the Okinawans. Although the Chinese had a friendly relationship with the Ryukyu Kingdom before its annexation by Japan, the denizens of the Ryukyu Kingdom were nevertheless non-Chinese to them. The relationship between the two was simply that of a tax collector and taxpayer. During the Qing Dynasty, before the Japanese annexation, the Ryukyu Kingdom had paid tributes to both China and Japan. It was dually subordinate to both countries; in other words, she served two masters. So just how much trust would the Chinese have been expected to extend to the Ryukyu people? Would they have revealed their national defense system to them? The Ryukyu kingdom officially became a part of Japan in 1879, but to the Ryukyu citizens, and to the Chinese who had migrated there as early as 1392, the Japanese were nothing more than invaders. Consequently, one must wonder just what the odds would have been that they would have revealed the true secrets of their national martial arts to their occupiers? When forced, they probably showed them the most basic movements and the simplest what-you-see-is-what-you-get version of their arts; that is, some basic stances, punches, and kicks. Some may have even given them a diluted version of some of their arts, so as to throw the foreigners off track.

The Japanese have always been a highly regimented and formal people. These attributes have been a part of their culture since before the days of the Samurai, and such character traits are still evident today in their family, school, and work culture. By way of contrast, the Chinese, being made up of many different ethnic groups, have always been fragmented, relatively less-formal, and disorderly. However, as a result of such a multicultural environment and such varied characteristics, the Chinese spirit grew to become amazingly creative, and would go on to invent (among many other things) paper, gunpowder, and many types of martial arts.

There exists an old axiom that states, "you never give your enemy the knife he needs to cut your throat," and when you consider that martial art was the Chinese means of defending themselves and their country, I consider it highly unlikely that the Chinese would ever teach non-Chinese the totality of their martial arts methods. I recall that Bruce Lee once opined that the Chinese martial arts were the ancestor of all of the Asian arts, predating Karate, Jujitsu, and Judo. It was his belief that other martial arts, such as Karate, were developed during the occupation of China by Japan, and that the Japanese assimilated what they were able to learn from the Chinese regarding such things as striking, throwing and grappling and then arranging these various techniques into a very workable formalized system. They ditched many of the forms of Chinese martial arts and created their own based upon certain Chinese martial art techniques. The result was a what-you-see-is-what-you-get series of katas that conformed to the Japanese culture and rituals (such as the Kabuki dance). They also implemented a uniform (gi) and (belt) ranking component into their system, which came from the influence of the military at the time.

It should be kept firmly in mind that the Chinese, being a naturally suspicious and secretive people, did not even teach their own people openly and freely. They kept their martial arts as family secrets, revealing only the best for the most trusted and capable family members. The forms were called Taolu (套路), meaning, "the path to the system." They were not referred to as "patterns," or Kata (型), like the Japanese did with their forms, but a way of thoroughly understanding the system that was being taught.

The Chinese have traditionally practiced their martial arts secretly, informally, and creatively. They didn't wear uniforms; just the clothes they would normally wear every day. They've never had a ranking system in their arts, but called each other only by family hierarchal titles, such as "elder brother," "younger brother," "father," or "uncle." However, because of this secrecy, many of the Chinese arts died with the masters who didn't choose an heir to their particular art. They may have felt that no one was worthy of inheriting or representing their art or some may have chosen an heir, but for whatever reason didn't reveal the totality of the art or system, thus the art that was passed down was incomplete. Moreover, those who were fortunate enough to have inherited an art may not have fully understood it, and consequently passed down a diluted version of it to the next generation. Then there were those who did not inherit the art or even learn the complete system, but falsified their credentials and taught incomplete and bastardized versions of the art. As a result, over many decades, many Chinese martial arts became flowery, ineffective, and disrespected, whereas the Japanese arts flourished because of the simple what-you-see-is-what-you-get product, their formal and systematic approach, and their disdain for fanciful and ineffective fighters. With the advent of the American presence in Japan after World War II, the Japanese martial arts were introduced to the West, and in time became supplemental sports to Western boxing and wrestling for American participants. With the formation of Japanese and American martial arts associations, along with well-organized exhibitions and marketing, the Japanese martial arts grew to become tremendously popular worldwide.

As compared with the rapid ascent in popularity of the Japanese martial arts since their inception, the Chinese martial arts have had a rather turbulent history. They reached their peak during the Ming Dynasty, but started to erode when the Manchurians from the North conquered China and established their own Qing Dynasty. The Chinese citizens, who were known as "Han" in those days, were banned from carrying any weapons and even from practicing their martial arts. The best of them were given high positions in the court and hired to teach the Manchurian royalty and officials. In essence they were highly paid to betray their own people. However, many of them taught a watered-down version of their arts, or else they modified them to become less efficient and deadly. Meanwhile, the defeated Chinese generals and soldiers continued practicing secretly and forming insurgency groups against the Manchurians. The Qing Dynasty ruled China for three hundred years. Although the Han Chinese and Manchurians eventually became one people, there were always small pockets of revolutionaries who wanted to oust the Qing Dynasty and revive the Ming Dynasty.

By the late nineteenth century the Qing Dynasty had begun to lose power to Western Imperialism. The ruler at the time, the Empress Dowager, spent the nation's funds extravagantly on both her palace and herself, leaving little left over for the army and navy, thus weakening her country's defense. China became no match against foreign troops in battles such as the First and Second Opium Wars. With each loss, the country suffered unfavorable peace treaties such as the one that allowed Britain to import opium into China, and another one that gave away China's vital seaports and cities to foreign powers. The citizens, particularly the Han Chinese, had grown hostile to the Empress Dowager's mismanagement of the country and of the Western imperialist presence, and insurgency groups again began to flourish. Some organizations fought for the ousting of both the Qing and foreign occupation, while others cohered with the Empress Dowager to oust only the foreign occupation. These rebel leaders and members of the insurgency groups came largely from secret martial arts societies; others were just merchants and peasants that were recruited. Pockets of insurgencies and Triads began breaking out everywhere in the country, the most significant being the Boxer Rebellion in Beijing. It is said that the Empress Dowager secretly supported and encouraged the rebels to fight the foreign powers while publicly denouncing the uprisings.

THE RISE (AND FALL) OF THE BOXERS

"The Boxer Rebellion," a phrase minted by Western historians, was referred to by the Chinese of the time as "the Righteous Harmony Society's Movement." It occurred over a three-year period (between 1898 to 1901), with the main incident occurring in June of 1900 in Beijing, when the "boxers" rampaged and killed both foreign and Chinese Christians. Foreign diplomats, soldiers, and expatriates, along with Chinese Christians took refuge at the Legation Quarter and the North Cathedral in Beijing. The boxers besieged the two premises from the outside.

In response, an alliance formed between eight foreign nations—Japan, Russia, Britain, France, the United States, Germany, Austria-Hungary, and Italy—to relieve the besieged colonists. Fifty-four ships, five thousand marines, and nearly fifty thousand soldiers were dispatched to quell the boxers. In August 1900, the Allied forces invaded and occupied Beijing. It became obvious very quickly that swords, spears and martial arts were no match for guns and cannons, as thousands of boxers died in the battles.

To prove to the Western powers her disapproval and disassociation from the boxers, the Empress Dowager captured the remaining boxers and beheaded them in a mass execution for the foreign diplomats to witness. The public executions served two purposes for her; first, it washed her hands of involvement with the Boxer Rebellion; second, it eliminated the Han Chinese insurgency once and for all. What was left of the best martial artists in Beijing and other parts of northern China were eliminated. Other rebels with martial arts skills suffered the same fate nationwide. (A 1963 Hollywood movie, *55 Days in Peking*, based on a book by Noel Gerson, sets the three main characters, played by Charlton Heston, Ava Gardner, and David Niven, in this historical background.)

On her deathbed in 1908 the Empress Dowager appointed her two-year-old nephew, Puyi, to become the new Emperor of China. However, an unstoppable revolution had already begun that would result in the demise of China's monarchy and launch the beginning of a republican government. The person who spearheaded this revolution was Sun Yatsen. After organizing many unsuccessful uprisings against the Qing Dynasty, Sun Yatsen's Xinhai Revolution finally overthrew it. He founded the Republic of China, and was elected as its provisional president by the provincial representatives on January 1, 1912. However, on March 10, General Yuan Shikai was given the position as a reward for getting Emperor Puyi to abdicate his throne.

Although the Qing Dynasty had fallen and the international community now officially recognized the Republic of China, much of the country was under the rule of warlords who each wanted to establish himself as the new emperor of China, including General Yuan Shikai. The governing members of the Republic of China were split in their support for Sun Yatsen and Yuan Shikai. Sun Yatsen had been the co-founder of the Kuomintang (the Chinese National Party), which eventually won the majority of seats in the Chinese parliament in 1913. Sun's Kuomintang army then attempted to overthrow Yuan, but failed. Sun escaped to Japan, and Yuan proclaimed himself the official Emperor of China in 1915.

Sun eventually returned to China in 1917 and started a military government in 1921 with the hope of unifying China through military conquest. He chose General Chiang Kaishek to be the commander of the National Revolutionary Army (NRA) and allied himself with the Communist Party of China. However, he never lived to see a unified China, dying on March 12, 1925. Chiang married Sun's sister-in-law, and established himself as the leader of the Kuomintang party.

Chiang Kaishek led his army along with the Communist army on the Northern Expedition, which eliminated both Yuan's army and his empire. Chiang then made himself the leader of China and severed its alliance with the Communists in 1927. Thus began five waves of besieging and massacring campaigns against the Communists; however, four of these resulted in defeat by Mao Zedong's Red Army. The last one involved one million Kuomintang soldiers, which drove Mao's Red Army on the famous eight thousand-mile Long March, from southeast China to northwest. However, the two parties allied again in 1937, when the Japanese invaded China.

The Communist guerrilla army, under the leadership of Mao Zedong, was instrumental in defeating the Japanese in China. When Japan eventually surrendered in 1945, the Kuomintang and the Chinese Communist Party of China (CCP) unsuccessfully tried to negotiate a coalition government. When it failed, the civil war resumed. The United States supported Chiang and supplied military assistance to his Kuomintang army against Mao. However, Mao's army proved to be the more disciplined, unified, and determined. They defeated Chiang's army, and took control of his last holdout in Chengdu, Sichuan in December 1949. Chiang escaped with his entourage to Taiwan. Under the leadership of Mao, China was finally unified after twenty years of international and civil wars. Mao became the Chairman of the Communist Party of the People's Republic of China.

The reason for this brief history lesson is that it is vitally important to understand the history of China to truly understand the history of Chinese martial arts. During these turbulent years of war, the reality was that no one had the time to engage in the practice of martial arts, as China was being perpetually bombed, invaded, and occupied by the Japanese. The citizens, martial artists included, were raped and massacred. There was a huge shortage of food and drinking water. If the Chinese people didn't die from the war, they died from starvation and dehydration. When Mao became the leader of the People's Republic of China in 1949 he implemented the Land Reform, which nationalized all privately owned properties. Land was taken from landlords and given to peasants. Millions of landlords, wealthy merchants, religious leaders and their congregations, Kuomintang members and soldiers, and political opponents were either publically executed or beaten to death. Those who survived were sent to labor camps for "reeducation." Historically, martial arts in China were only practiced by the upper- and middle classes, since the poor were only concerned with their own day-to-day struggles to survive. There is an old Chinese dictum that says, "The poor studies literature, but the rich plays martial arts." As a result, most of China's martial artists were in this group of wealthy landlords and merchants, therefore, were either executed or persecuted.

Between the years 1959 to 1962 an unsuccessful campaign to boost agriculture and industry was followed by natural disasters that killed or starved an estimated thirty million Chinese people. During this era the Chinese citizens were rationed one kilogram of meat per year per person, and one liter of cooking oil per person per year. You can be certain that no one was practicing Tai Chi in the parks or pounding on Ip Man's wooden dummy in Foshan (Fatsan) during this period.

All private property became nationalized. Houses and apartments were communized, with large properties being occupied by several families or made into commune offices. There was no such thing as one house for one family or one bedroom for one person. It was one room for one family. Everything in the house was shared—a commune leader made sure of that. Knowing this, it is almost impossible to conceive that a human-sized martial arts training device such as a wooden dummy would have existed in a commune household shared by several families. It would have better served as firewood for cooking or heating a Chinese family's house in the winter.

In 1966, Mao saw and feared that the revolution was replacing the old bourgeois class with a new ruling class; therefore, he and his wife implemented the *Cultural Revolution*, banning any practice of traditional culture such as ancestor or deity worship, martial arts, classical opera, music, dances, or anything else that was associated with the old China. He encouraged the citizens to police each other, causing children to accuse their parents of breaking the law—the result of which pitted neighbor against neighbor. Young people formed policing and tribunal groups they called the "Red Guards." The Red Guards ran amok, destroying ancient temples, old artifacts, and schools. They then began the persecution of educators and intellectuals, banishing them to the countryside for hard labor and reeducation. The practice of religion, traditional philosophy, and culture were also banned. So, you can be sure that there weren't any Buddhist monks or Taoists practicing martial arts or meditating inside the Shaolin or Wudang temples during this period.

When the Chinese Communist Party (CCP) first took power in 1949 they banned all martial arts for fear of a revolution. Chinese history is full of revolutions that were instigated by martial artists, so to ensure that this didn't happen again, the CCP's solution was to obliterate them. The Cultural Revolution, which started in 1966, hammered the last nail onto the coffin of the Chinese martial arts, in what was probably the lowest point for Chinese martial arts in the history of China.

When Mao eventually died in 1976, China began to change under the leadership of Deng Xiaoping and most of Mao's Cultural Revolution reforms were abandoned by 1978. However, the citizens were fearful and suspicious of new reforms, lest they should change again, and no one wanted to be exposed to further persecution. As a result, during the 1980s the Chinese people conducted themselves as if the Cultural Revolution was still in effect. It wasn't until the CCP officially declared that all of the ancient Chinese traditions, religions and martial arts practices that were under government control would now be legal that people started to feel comfortable about practicing them. The Government began to re-allow the celebration of some traditional festivals by designating those days as holidays. It returned properties that had been seized by the state back to their rightful owners, but with the proviso that the land itself remained state-owned. It allowed the return of religion—providing that the religion met with government approved (and selected) religious leaders; the government rejected leaders from outside of China, such as the Pope in Rome or the Dalai Lama in Dharamsala. It selected representatives for martial arts but they were encouraged to remove the fighting aspect from their arts, revising them for health and exhibition purposes only. The government oversaw the creation of a new art called Wushu, and then simplified the Tai Chi forms, placing the emphasis on the art's health promoting properties rather than its fighting component.

With the popularity of Hong Kong action movies (even Mao was said to have been a fan of Bruce Lee's movies), the Chinese Government began producing them also, the earliest and most popular one being *The Shaolin Temple*, starring a young Jet Li, who had won several national Wushu forms competitions.

It was only when the Government had opened the doors of China to the West, and particularly to the revenue generated by tourism, that they realized that there was a significant market for martial arts and cultural tourism. As a result they began to resurrect and renovate the temples throughout China that had been destroyed and neglected, especially those that had a deep martial arts history like the northern Shaolin Temple. And, with the arrival of Western martial-arts tourists, many Chinese martial-arts "masters" suddenly surfaced. But where did they come from? How did they survive Mao's persecution? How did they survive the famine and starvation that had beset the country? How did they survive the Cultural Revolution? How, where, and when did they practice their martial arts diligently enough to achieve "master" status? Who were their masters? How did their masters survive? Where did they dig up people with any knowledge of Buddhism to fill the temples after eradicating both the religion and its practitioners since 1949?

The truth of the matter is that those who were not killed or persecuted before and immediately after the Communist takeover of China had escaped to Hong Kong, Macau, Taiwan, Southeast Asia, and to the West. These refugees were the ones who truly preserved the Chinese culture and Chinese martial arts. It was through these individuals that the Chinese martial arts came to be known today throughout the world. They may not have been the best of China's martial artists, but they were the ones who kept the traditions alive, and passed the various Chinese martial arts on to the next generations.

With Chinese martial arts so shrouded in mystery and so many of its masters dying in war and revolution, many forms of Chinese martial arts died with them. This is why there are so many ineffective Chinese fighting arts today. It surely didn't help matters having the Chinese Communist Party stamp out martial arts for forty years and then reviving them solely for the purpose of commercialization.

Having said all this, I must say that the Chinese are resilient people. In just thirty years, they've raised themselves from Third-World status to one of the three most powerful countries in the world in terms of its economy, military, and Olympic athletes. So, it is not surprising that they've also raised their status in martial arts in these three decades—particularly in Tai Chi. However, there is no denying that there was a period in modern China where martial art was at its lowest point. Chen Tai Chi Grandmaster Feng Zhiqiang, who passed away in 2012, admitted how this period stifled his growth in martial arts and deprived him of the goals he could have achieved. There were only a few masters like him in China who were able to pick up from where they had left off before martial arts were banned, but in most cases, others who survived execution, persecution, starvation, illness, and even death from old age, lost interest in carrying on their martial arts training.

To our great fortune, however, some great masters did escape and survive the Chinese wars and revolutions. One such master was my Great-Grandmaster Ip Man, who escaped to Hong Kong in 1949 before the complete takeover of China by the Communist Party.

FOUR

GRANDMASTER IP MAN

G REAT-GRANDMASTER IP MAN WAS but one of a handful of top martial artists who escaped the wrath of the Chinese wars and the Communist genocides. To be certain, there were others who escaped to neighboring countries, some of whom even landed on the shores of Europe and America. However, no one has made as much impact on Chinese martial arts in the eyes of the international martial arts community. Indeed, the only person who has surpassed him in fame was his student, Bruce Lee. These two legends are almost synonymous with each other, as Bruce Lee may not have become who he was if not for Ip Man, and Ip Man may not have become as famous today had it not been for Bruce Lee.

Great-Grandmaster Ip Man was an unassuming, modest, and humble man. The last thing he would have wanted was today's media attention and he certainly was not the grandiose character the Ip Man movies have made him out to be. I will not go into Ip Man's biography since much has been written about him elsewhere, and because I possess no first hand information about him. However, I will state a few things that I had heard about him when I was practicing Wing Chun before he died (I started my Wing Chun training in 1970; Ip Man died in 1972).

According to my sources, who knew him personally, he was a very conservative Chinese man. He grew up in China at a time when it was crumbling under the rule of the Manchurians and the occupation of foreign powers. It has been estimated that one-third of the then Chinese population was addicted to the opium that was brought in by the British under the Unequal

Treaty Act, and which was forced upon the Manchurian government after several unsuccessful battles against importing it. The Chinese race became known throughout the Asian world as the "Sick Man of Asia"—a label and stigma that every Chinese hated and wanted to get rid of. You may recall this phrase as being an insult leveled by the Japanese at the Chinese martial artists in Bruce Lee's second film *The Chinese Connection* (released as *Fist of Fury* in Europe and Asia).

In 1908, at the age of fifteen, Ip Man went to Hong Kong to study at St. Stephen's College, which was then a British program school that had been established only five years before. The college was built exclusively for the children of expatriates and Chinese elites. Hong Kong, at the time, was already under the rule of the British Government, as China had lost Hong Kong to Britain during the First Opium War in 1842.

Both in the school and in Hong Kong Ip Man had experienced discrimination from foreign students and the British establishment. When he returned to Foshan (Fatsan in Cantonese), China, nine years later he carried with him feelings of suspicion and intense dislike for all Westerners. Such feelings were only augmented by the Japanese occupation of China during the Second World War.

In China, Ip Man's family was wealthy and he worked as a police officer for the Kuomintang government. Even in those early days he had acquired a reputation for being an extremely skilled martial artist. It was these three factors that automatically placed him in the crosshairs for execution or imprisonment when the Chinese Communist Party took control of China in 1949. As a result, his choice was simple: escape China or die. Although he had no love for the British, Hong Kong was probably his only choice because he had friends there and he could communicate in his native dialect—Cantonese—which was spoken widely in Hong Kong.

He lived in Hong Kong from 1949 until his death in 1972. As early as 1949, the Hong Kong population, especially the middle and upper classes, had given up Chinese attire, and were then in the custom of wearing Western suits. Doing so was considered a show of class, education, and modernization. By the 1960s, even the poor population of Hong Kong had switched to Western clothing; if they didn't wear suits, they at least wore Western shirts, pants and shoes. However, Ip Man continued wearing traditional Chinese attire, in spite of being educated in a British school during his youth. He was making a statement by doing so. He was proud of his culture and heritage, and was unwilling to bend his knee to the false and transient idols of fashion, modernization, and Western influence. There were others from other cultures before him that did likewise. Gandhi, the great Indian leader, who had even acquired a law degree in London and

Grandmaster IP Man

was well aware of the status of wearing a Western suit, chose instead to wear traditional Indian attire upon his return to India and the start of his campaign to free the country from British rule. He even wore the "dhoti" (Indian loincloth) and shawl to meet King George V and Queen Mary at Buckingham Palace.

To Ip Man the art of Wing Chun was a part of his Chinese cultural heritage. He considered it to be a Chinese treasure and the supreme self-defense system. He did not want to share it with the West for fear of it becoming diluted, or for fear of it being used against the Chinese people. When he first learned Wing Chun as a young boy in Foshan, he trained with only a handful of practitioners. Later when he started teaching the art, he also restricted his class size to only a handful of students and did it only on a part-time basis. Wing Chun had always been taught that way, as it is an art that requires the development of highly refined tactile sensory skills, which can only be properly taught by a skillful practitioner and teacher through hand-to-hand contact. In addition, Wing Chun was meant to be kept secret, divulged only to one's most trusted family members and friends. Ip Man never thought of making a career out of it and neither did any of his Wing Chun forebears.

Like many others, he left his family and wealth behind in Foshan to go to Hong Kong in 1949. His situation in Hong Kong now stood in big contrast to what he had experienced in the past. For one thing he was now fifty-six years old. He didn't have any trade skills (his martial art skills were not considered valuable in those days) nor work experience, other than being a policeman in Foshan. His disdain for the British occupation of Hong Kong probably prevented him from even applying for a police job there. However, his friends were able to secure a job for him at a restaurant where he shared a room with other workers. He was able to make new friends through the Hong Kong Restaurant Workers' Association, which also had a club for martial artists, headed by a man named Leung Seung. Ip Man did not let on to anyone that he was a martial artist. Being a small and unassuming man, no one even suspected.

In order to pass the time Ip Man attended the martial arts classes, but primarily just for the social intercourse. However, on one occasion when Leung Seung was conducting his class, Ip Man couldn't help but snicker at what Leung Seung was doing with his students. This was taken as an insult and prompted Leung Seung to invite Ip Man to stand up and exchange hands with him, with the intent of "teaching him a lesson." Ip Man at first declined, but the crowd, in jest, cheered and jeered him to take up the challenge for their entertainment. Believing Leung Seung to be not much of a challenge, Ip Man stood up. He was only 5'3" (160 centimeters) and weighed

[29]

no more than 135 pounds (61 kilograms), while Leung Seung stood 5' 7" (170 centimeters), and weighed around 170 pounds (77 kilograms).

The comic situation that the crowd had expected turned out to be exactly that; only the role of the players was the opposite of what they had envisioned. Ip Man easily and effortlessly overpowered Leung Seung in just a few moves. Only then did Leung Seung and the crowd realize the level of skill and knowledge that Ip Man possessed. Leung Seung immediately asked to become Ip Man's student, and relinquished his position as the chief instructor. Great-Grandmaster Ip Man accepted Leung Seung as his first student, and later reluctantly accepted the position of chief instructor of martial arts for the Hong Kong Restaurant Workers' Association, after repeated pleas from its members.

When he began teaching at the Association in the 1950s his students consisted primarily of restaurant workers who were both poor and poorly educated. It must have been difficult for him to communicate the deeper ideology of Wing Chun to them, but he made the attempt with each class that he taught, despite being unaccustomed to teaching large classes. However, by the 1960s, he was becoming known outside of the Association community, and was attracting wealthier and better-educated students to his classes who could better comprehend the deeper underpinnings of his art. With their support, he established the Ving Tsun Athletic Association.

Ip Man's Wing Chun evolved through a lengthy process of trial and error. Consequently, he taught differently from one decade to another. Although many came through his schools, only a few were given private lessons, and fewer still were able to grasp the deeper understanding of Wing Chun he was attempting to communicate. Although there were many members in the Association who joined his Wing Chun classes, only a few of them were truly dedicated and took the art seriously enough to train regularly and stay the course until Great-Grandmaster Ip Man's passing. Some who come to mind are Leung Seung, Lok Yiu, Chu Shongtin, Wong Shun Leung and Moy Yat. Many came and went. Some were just young men who would soon leave Hong Kong to attend school overseas. One of these young men was an individual by the name of Bruce Lee.

ENTER THE LITTLE DRAGON

Bruce Lee's rare martial arts talent was a super-quick muscular reflex. Although he had just a few years of Wing Chun training, Lee was able to grasp the essence of the art quickly; through dedication and diligent practice he was able to develop himself over time into a truly superior and unique martial artist. This can't be said about other teenagers who left Hong Kong and their Wing Chun training after just a few years of instruction.

I find it hard to believe that some of the other teenagers who left Hong Kong at the age of seventeen or eighteen at that time can claim to have had closed-door training sessions with the then sixty-five year-old Ip Man. Grandmasters like Leung Seung, Lok Yiu, Chu Shong Tin, Wong Shun Leung, and Moy Yat never made such claims in spite of training (and having a close relationship) with the Great-Grandmaster until his death. Even if they received private lessons, they never broadcasted it. The closest that Bruce Lee got to a private lesson was when he claimed to have fooled other students into thinking that the class was cancelled, so that when they went home he was able to study one-on-one with his teacher (who, during his final year and a half in Hong Kong was Wong Shun Leung). This story, if true, might have happened once, as nobody would have fallen for it the next time. They would all have known about it by the next day and Great-Grandmaster Ip Man would not have taken it lightly. Indeed, when my co-author John Little spoke with Ip Man's eldest son Ip Chun about this in 2009, he was told, "If Bruce Lee had misbehaved like this it would have been surprising to Ip Man. If it were true then Ip Man wouldn't have known about it. If he knew about it, he definitely would have scolded him. Bruce Lee was successful because he was determined. He studied at Dai Kok Chuy (St. Josephs), near Ip Man's home, and my father told me that Lee would get out of school at 3:00 pm, carrying his schoolbag, walking and practicing his Kung Fu while he walked. So this dedication to the art is what led to him being so successful. He was very dedicated."

If Ip Man was in the habit of conducting closed-door sessions, Bruce Lee would most certainly have been included because, coming from a well-to-do family, he could have afforded the private lessons. However, Lee never claimed to have had closed-door sessions with the master; unfortunately, some of his peers have made these unfounded claims.

Bruce Lee was an exceptionally talented martial artist. He dedicated his life fully to it. He had the looks, personality, physique and charisma to succeed in the film world. He fed the West what they've always admired: speed, strength, and showmanship. The United States, and particularly Hollywood, propelled Lee to international superstardom. Before that, Lee had already established himself as a martial arts icon in Asia. It was almost inevitable that he should become world-renowned. Bruce Lee wanted fame, and he worked hard to achieve it. GGM Ip Man didn't want fame, but he got it anyway. He didn't even want Wing Chun to become a famous art; he simply wanted Wing Chun to be preserved—and then only for the Chinese people. From today's perspective, this may not sound politically correct, but based on the personal experience and history, one should understand the context that underlay his position. He had seen and experienced Chinese people being bullied by foreigners; he had witnessed the Chinese martial arts stolen, corrupted, and rebranded by other nationalities. He simply would not contribute to the continuation of such a trend. His character was such that he simply wouldn't allow it.

Ip Man retired from teaching by the mid nineteen sixties. However, he authorized and attended the inauguration of various Wing Chun schools that were opened by his senior students in Hong Kong and Kowloon, which he enjoyed visiting from time to time. He was diagnosed with throat cancer in 1970 and his health began to deteriorate gradually. Finally, he passed away at the age of 79. He bequeathed to us both a legacy and a gift that we now enjoy thoroughly. However, something went terribly wrong over the years since then; his art has become controversial, with practitioners bickering amongst each other as to who possesses the purest form.

One thing very strange about this whole scenario is that as traditional as he was, and although he had a considerable amount of time to ponder the situation, he did not select an heir to his legacy. Traditionally, every master of a martial art would select and groom a disciple to represent and inherit his art. He would choose a person not only for his skills, but also for his character, intelligence, and principles. Was it because he did not see anyone fit for the role or had he decided that the art itself requires a personal journey of comprehension and self-mastery that each student must make on his own? Certainly there would appear to be individuals within those groups who were immensely worthy and very talented in the art—at least in judging the situation from the outside. Immediately after his death some shamefully proclaimed themselves to be his heir; however, the truth was too obvious for the Wing Chun community to accept such proclamations. Today, there is no one person who represents the art of Wing Chun universally, and the dispute goes on.

Perhaps this is why GGM Ip Man didn't want Wing Chun to be spread worldwide. I'm grateful that I was able to learn Wing Chun because he had taught it openly. Great-Grandmaster Ip Man did not pass down a sport but an art, culture, tradition, and treasure. For this reason I am morally obliged to do my best to preserve it in its original state, including the history that came with it. To modify it would be disrespectful to Ip Man, the original founders of the art, and the art itself. This is not to say that I treat every word Ip Man said as God's truth, but I do believe that he spoke and taught truthfully.

FIVE

ON THE ORIGIN OF WING CHUN

In one of the few interviews Ip Man ever gave during his life, a Hong Kong newspaperman asked him about the origins of Wing Chun. In reply, he related a story that is now commonly known amongst Wing Chun practitioners and the general public. He later wrote it down upon a scroll and assigned his student Moy Yat to inscribe it in stone. I will not go into the details but it does bring up some rather important points that are under debate these days.

IP MAN'S STORY OF WING CHUN

According to Ip Man there once was an abbess named Ng Mui in the Shaolin Temple in Henan, who was a skilled martial artist. When the Manchurians set fire to the temple and attacked it, she escaped to the White Crane Temple in Daliang Mountain that bordered the Yunnan and Sichuan provinces. There, she met a girl named Yim Wing Chun and her father, who were selling tofu at the bottom of the mountain.

Wing Chun's father was accused of a crime he did not commit in Guangzhou, in Guangdong province, and so he fled, taking Wing Chun with him to southwest China. Once there, a local warlord became interested in Wing Chun, and made every attempt to force her into marrying him. Wing Chun sought refuge at the White Crane Temple, where the abbess Ng Mui began training her in a new martial art that she had recently developed. After training Wing Chun for some time, Ng Mui felt that Wing Chun was ready to defend herself against the warlord. When the warlord attempted to take Wing Chun away by force, Wing Chun defeated him in a public fight. The warlord was so shamed by the defeat that he ran away, and was never seen again.

Later, Wing Chun married Leung Bokchao (in Guangzhou), who was also a skilled martial artist. Together they further developed the art and systematized it; Leung Bokchao then christened the newly developed art after his wife and the art of "Wing Chun" was born. Later the husband and wife taught their martial art to friends who were actors in the Red Junk Opera, and who, in turn, taught it to others, including Dr. Leung Jan in Foshan (Fatsan). Dr. Leung taught Chan Wah Shun, who later would take Ip Man as his last student. The rest, as they say, is history. However, Ip Man's version of the history of the art of Wing Chun has recently come under criticism.

Some researchers are now claiming that there were no such personages as Ng Mui, Yim Wing Chun, or Leung Bokchao, and that the art of Wing Chun began at the Shaolin Temple and was further developed by anti-Qing insurgents who posed as actors in the Red Junk Opera troupe. It is claimed that they concocted the story about Yim Wing Chun to throw off the Manchurian insurgent-hunters. Yet another recent version claims that a deadly form of Wing Chun was developed by a secret gangster society called the Black Flag, and that they passed down a milder version to the Red Flag group, which found its way to Great-Grandmaster Ip Man.

To the critics of GGM Ip Man's version I have to ask, "Where did all of this information that you base your version of the art's origin come from?" It certainly couldn't have come from China, as the martial arts had at this point in time been inactive for more than forty years. It appears to me that this new information comes from the mouths of practitioners who weren't even born when the Chinese Communist Party took control of China in 1949, or even during the Cultural Revolution from 1966 to 1978. They are merely opinions from people who have come to Wing Chun quite recently. If they were forty years old at the time they were interviewed in 2010, they would have been born in 1970—in the thick of the Cultural Revolution. If they started learning martial arts in 1990, when they were twenty, who were their masters? How old were these masters in 1990? If they were forty years old, they would have been born in 1950, and perhaps learned Wing Chun when they were twenty years old in 1970—which puts them right in the thick of the Cultural Revolution when the martial arts were fully banned throughout China. Who were their masters? Great-Grandmaster Ip Man's peers? Those who survived Sun Yatsen's revolution, the Japanese invasion, World War II, the civil war, and the Chinese Communist Party's massacre of the elite? If the wars and famine didn't kill them, they would have died from old age around 1972 just as GGM Ip Man did at the age of seventy-nine. Even if they lived to be a hundred years old, that would bring them to about 1999. And yet all of this information came out after the year 2000.

While it is true that it takes but one surviving martial artist with knowledge of his art's history to pass the information on orally to the next generation, when there are different versions of the oral history one must examine the plausibility through probable deduction. For example, let's consider for a moment the story of the revolutionists posing as actors in the Red Junk Opera troupe. They were opera actors during the day and fought at night as masked marauders, while traveling on the river systems from town to town; or perhaps they acted in the evenings and fought during the day. What would the troupe do when one or more of them were killed while fighting the Manchurians? The Red Junk Opera actors were not just some second-rate thespians; they were highly trained from childhood to perform difficult acrobatics, dances, and classical roles. They'd be booed off the stage and given no audience at all if some insurgents simply posed as actors. Moreover, some of these actors had to play female roles in the operas; this required real acting skills. A poseur's true identity would soon be discovered as a result of his poor acting skills. Even if they were true actors who took part in the insurgency, how would it help if they told the Manchurian captors that they inherited their martial art from a woman?

As for the Black Flag society, they would have been smoked out and slaughtered by the Chinese Communist Party within the first month of their rule. The Party viewed secret societies, corrupt officials, and elite classes as the axis of evil that brought the country down prior to their rule. No secret society member would have survived to tell any story about the Black or Red Flag societies today. Admitting any connection to any secret society in the past would have landed them in prison, if not on the execution block.

The newer versions of the history of Wing Chun tend to gain support owing to the fact that newcomers to Wing Chun find themselves at the bottom rung of the Ip Man lineage. Some find dissatisfaction from the school they're in or the teacher they're learning from, and earnestly seek for a better way and a higher truth. However, there are those whose egos can't accept where they are in the pecking order of the lineage of the art, and the temptation beckons to jump ranks by taking a two-week course with one of Ip Man's first generation students, which then allows them to claim to be one of his "second generation" students. Then there are those who are not happy with their second-generation ranking. They can't be GGM Ip Man's first generation student because he is no longer around, and so they look for someone in China or elsewhere who is not related to Ip Man's lineage, and become this new master's "first generation" student or representative—and this after only a few weeks of training! As long as the student promotes and builds up the new master's reputation, he will be not only be his first generation student, but also his best student!

This is far more common in the martial arts world than one might think at first blush. And this is only one class of lineage chaser; other classes involve people who make themselves Sijos—"great-great grandfathers" of an art simply by mixing techniques from various martial arts together and giving the hybrid product a new name. They no longer are under any masters, but become masters themselves; starting at a level higher than the sifus they originally learned from and even higher than their grandmasters. Sadly, this is the state that the art of Wing Chun is in today. These are the people who are going around disputing the veracity of Great-Grandmaster Ip Man's art of Wing Chun and its history.

Like most practitioners of Wing Chun, I, too, am deeply interested in its history, but I have no interest at all in the drama and the politics. I'm more interested in how it was actually developed. I have a hypothesis that I've developed over the decades from a long process of logical deduction and I think it is a more sound hypothesis than many of the ones that have been making the rounds recently. Although there is no question that the actors in the Red Junk Opera were involved in the development of Wing Chun, I don't believe that they were the founders of the art. Neither do I believe that the art was developed at the Shaolin Temple, nor by the Black Flag secret society.

If you look at other Chinese martial arts such as Shaolin, Tai Chi, Praying Mantis, White Crane, White Eyebrows, or Bagua, the family tree is clearly drawn showing the name of the founder (or at least the name of the one who put the art on the map), the names of the descendants, the name of the place it was developed, and the name of the art, which is usually associated with the founder, place, or theme of the art. To the Chinese, keeping a record of the family tree is of the utmost importance. I have a copy of my family tree going back sixteen generations before me. Had not China suffered all the wars that she did during the last three hundred years, I might have records going back even further. During China's Cultural Revolution, ancestor worship was outlawed. Keeping records of family trees, displaying pictures of ancestors in one's home, or even visiting them at gravesites would have landed a person either in prison or a labor camp. A family member of mine hid a handwritten record of our family history in a crack in the wooden stairs of his home and only took it out after the law was abolished in the 1980s. It was so important to him that he risked his life in preserving it.

If the Red Junk Opera actors were the true founders of Wing Chun, then there would have been a written or verbal record stating so. There is none.

Whatever record is available now is simply a list of names of people who were practitioners of the art. Similarly, if Wing Chun was developed within the Shaolin Temple, then it would probably have been named "Shaolin Fists." For that matter, there is a fighting system called Shaolin Fists, and it is nothing like Wing Chun conceptually or systematically. "New research" says that there was a room named "Eternal Spring" (永春) in the Shaolin Temple where a separate art was developed but I don't buy this at all. If a software house became contracted to develop a new and superior accounting program, wouldn't the developers work together to come up with the one product that they thought was the best? They wouldn't have two competing products under the banner of one company. Whatever programs they developed and tested, the best one would be the one they'd use as the "house system." If the group in the Eternal Spring hall came up with the best product, the senior abbots would have given it the thumbs up and branded it Shaolin Fists—not Eternal Spring Fists. In fact, as I mentioned, they did develop a Shaolin Fists system—and it doesn't resemble anything like Wing Chun.

The Shaolin Fists system is based on super-hard conditioning and requires extensive flexibility training of the human body. The thought being that if you toughen all parts of your body, including the head, throat and testicles, you'll not only be able to withstand the hardest hits, but also be able to carry on fighting until you subdue your foe. Moreover, you'll become so flexible that you will be able to twist, roll and bend away from all types of weapons attacks. You will toughen your arms and legs and hit like iron. Basically, you will become a superman—that is until you reach age 35, when your body can no longer take that kind of abuse and you're forced to retire and become a fat meditating monk. This represents a huge disparity between the philosophy of Wing Chun and Shaolin Fists, and I, at least, see no correlation at all between the two.

As for the Black Flag theory, I again see no correlation with Wing Chun. In all of martial arts history, there hasn't been any secret society that has founded or developed any martial art. Sure, there were many secret societies, but none that had a martial art associated with it. The gangsters wouldn't have had the interest, patience, or desire to do so. Secret societies, like the Mafia, the Triads, and the Russian Mobs today, are just interested in robbing society of its wealth, and to live life like kings. They don't need to develop any martial art when they can easily afford hit men. Why bother discussing Tansau, Bongsau, or Fooksau, or doing Chisau, in the courtyard when they could be having the wildest time at the whorehouse next door? Granted, some gang members may have trained in Wing Chun, but I can't believe that they had the intelligence and patience to develop such a fine and complex art.

So now that I've told you my reasons as to why I don't believe the revisionist's history of Wing Chun, I should throw my hat in the ring and give you my take on the origins of the art. There are Wing Chun practitioners who believe that Ip Man simply made up the story of Wing Chun's origin. Then there are those who believe Ip Man told it truthfully, but that he was only retelling what he himself had been told by his masters—which was a lie from the very beginning. Again, these hypotheses are being advanced by relative newcomers to the art of Wing Chun. However, I don't believe that Ip Man was a fool; he was well educated, humble, honest, and possessed of a high level of integrity and dignity—and he would have been intelligent enough to differentiate fact from fiction. The story of Yim Wing Chun meant enough for him to commission his student Moy Yat to etch it in stone.

From my forty-plus years of training, experience and understanding of Wing Chun, I have no doubt that the art is more conformed to a woman's structure and mindset than to that of a man's. For this reason, men tend to struggle to master the art or even to do well against martial artists from other systems today. Since Ip Man's departure, there hasn't been anyone as proficient as he was in Wing Chun. He was a small and gentle man. In fact, he became even more skillful in his senior years when he had lost muscle mass and his testosterone levels naturally declined. It's worthy to note that the best Wing Chun practitioner amongst the Red Junk Opera actors was a man named Leung Yitai, the person who played the female role on stage, and also the person who taught Dr. Leung Jan.

When you look at Wing Chun's horse (stance), Tansau, postures and concepts, they are all very strange and contradictory to male structure and thinking. Women have no obstacles between their legs, and so can comfortably press their knees inward (which is the basic stance in Wing Chun). Also, because of their proportionately wider pelvis compared to men, their femurs (thigh bones) verge naturally inward towards the knees, while men's femurs are more perpendicularly aligned.

Women can also execute a Tansau more easily and naturally because of their inherently inward-angled upper arms. If you don't believe me, ask your girlfriend or sister to fully stretch their arms out in front of them, with their palms touching at the baby-finger edge, and see how her forearms close the opening in the Centerline Plane. Women also have an inherently stronger and differently shaped lordosis (lower vertebrae) than males do in order to prepare them for childbirth. This gives women a stronger waist, posture and pelvis for better and stronger lower-trunk control.

As the saying goes, "Behind every great man, there is a great woman." An old-fashioned woman is happy to appear to take the backseat, because she knows that, in reality, she's at the forefront. It allows her to assuage a man's ego while still retaining overall control. Men are too assertive and direct, which often gets them into trouble. Women, by contrast, are more indirect and yielding, and yet stay atop. This is the mentality required in perfecting one's performance in Wing Chun.

It is interesting how in Ip Man's story, the Abbess Ng Mui is from Henan (some say from Fujian), and Yim Wing Chun from Guangdong—both in eastern China—yet they meet 2,000 kilometers away at the Daliang Mountain in Southwest China, then Yim Wing Chun returns all the way back to Guangdong where she and her husband develop the art further. A generation or two later, the art had found its way to Foshan, where Dr. Leung Jan, Chan Wah Shun, and Ip Man lived. I say "interesting" because Wing Chun is considered a southeastern Chinese martial art. If this were a made-up story, why make it so elaborate as to take Yim Wing Chun from Southeast China to Southwest China and then return her back to Southeast, when the story could have easily placed her in Southeast China to develop the art like other Chinese arts such as Hong Gar, Choy Layfat, Fujian White Crane, and Southern Shaolin?

I believe that there is great significance in this travel story. The most obvious one being that Abbess Ng Mui, Yim Wing Chun, and Yim Wing Chun's father were attempting to escape from the Manchurian soldiers. Where better to hide than 2,000 kilometers away from home? Remember, in those days there were no planes, trains or automobiles. It would have taken the Manchurian soldiers no less than four hundred days on foot and a hundred days on horse to travel across the country. It wouldn't have been logistically worthwhile for the Manchurian government to dispatch a small army across the country to hunt for just one or two criminals. In addition, the Daliang Mountain is situated at the border of Sichuan and Yunnan provinces in Southwest China. Yunnan particularly would have been a good hideout for Ng Mui and Wing Chun. Yunnan translates to "South of the Clouds" and it always was, and still is, considered a faraway, remote and inaccessible province in China. Until recently, the only means of traveling its narrow mountainous roads and torrential rivers was by mule, yak, sheep-skin floats, and rope-glides. Furthermore, Yunnan is inhabited by twenty-five major ethnic minorities and twenty-six minor indigenous groups; it was always ruled by fierce ethnic warlords whom the central government was never quite able to conquer, colonize, or enslave. Even in recent Chinese history it stands out as one of the last Chinese provinces to be converted to Communism. Because of its isolation from the rest of China, it was often used as a place of banishment for political exiles and fugitives.

Yunnan shares borders with Tibet (when it was an independent country), India, Nepal, Myanmar (Burma), Laos, and Vietnam. Any fugitive that had fled to Yunnan could easily sneak across into one of these countries without drawing attention; by contrast, an army couldn't do so without proper authorization. This was the last stronghold and passageway that Chiang Kaishek's Kuomintang remaining soldiers used to escape from the pursuing Red Army.

Although International maps show only one name for Daliang Mountain, the regional folks call the Sichuan section of the mountain Daliangshan (Large Cool Mountain), and the Yunnan section, Xiaoliangshan (Small Cool Mountain). I suspect that Abbess Ng Mui and Yim Wing Chun were on the Yunnan side of the Mountain because of its remoteness and close proximity to the borders of these other countries. Also, Yunnan was inhabited by hill tribes that were always unfriendly with the central government, whether Chinese or Manchurian.

Now let's consider another significant aspect of this cross-country travel. I doubt very much that a sophisticated and rich art like Wing Chun could have sprouted from the mere witnessing of a fight between a crane and a snake as some have claimed. I don't think it could have even been an inspiration to develop an art as rich as Wing Chun. In all my years of practice and teaching, neither my teachers nor I have ever referenced the crane or snake for any Wing Chun movement. In fact, Ip Man's written account of the origins of Wing Chun never mentioned Abbess Ng Mui witnessing a crane fighting a snake or fox. The crane, snake, and fox story appears to have surfaced later, somehow, from somewhere else. Also, a fighting system is not developed overnight in a dream or by a sighting. It has been said that Abbess Ng Mui was already a skilled Shaolin martial artist. It has also been said that Ng Mui found both the Shaolin art and training unsuitable for her feminine stature. If that was the case, why did she not develop a female fighting system while she was still at the Shaolin Temple? If she did, and such a system had proven sufficient to overpower the Shaolin fighters, it would have become a Shaolin art on the spot with every monk practicing it thereafter. The story of Wing Chun would have been a very simple one—just saying that it was developed at the Shaolin Temple would have sufficed instead of taking Ng Mui to Southwest China where she is somehow enlightened to create a new system and teach it to Yim Wing Chun, who then brings it back to Southeast China. If someone wanted to lie about the origin of Wing Chun, he wouldn't need to make it so elaborate, unless he was a child or a poor liar.

I believe Ip Man's version of the history of Wing Chun over any of the others that have surfaced over the years because it came from a man of integrity. I have also looked for evidence for his story, and have found more than enough to satisfy my intellectual curiosity. But let me tell you something that you may not know; in the Yunnan side of Daliang Mountain, called Xiaoliang, there is a village located by a lake called Lugu. It is inhabited by an indigenous tribe called the Mosuo. What is unique about this tribe is that it is a matriarchal one. In other words, its women are the heads of the families and of the tribe. They don't have traditional marriages, per se, but have what they call "walking marriages." Men do not live with the women; they only come at night and leave before dawn. The men possess no rights to property or the children they father. (Read more about it at www.ethnic-china.com/Moso/mosomarriage.htm.) The Lugu Lake Village still exists today, and the Mosuo people are still operating on a matriarchal system. They are thought to be a spinoff from the Tibetan people, and have been around for at least a thousand years. Apart from the Mosuo tribe, there exist other matriarchal and semi-matriarchal tribes in Yunnan, Sichuan, and the neighboring countries such as Myanmar, Laos, Cambodia and Thailand.

In a matriarchal society, where women are property owners, heads of families and leaders of villages, wouldn't it stand to reason that they would have had a self-defense system in place? Wouldn't the patriarchal villages in the vicinity have been a threat to them? Wouldn't the matriarchal villages have empowered fellow women to protect their village (instead of men) to maintain their matriarchal system? And wouldn't they then have had to develop a unique fighting system suitable for women, particularly one that had proven capable of defeating men?

Abbess Ng Mui and Yim Wing Chun came from Southeast China, where women were dainty and submissive, and where men treated them like property, trading and selling them at will. My theory is that Abbess Ng Mui must have come across a matriarchal village, and saw these powerful women at work. Abbess Ng Mui, already being a fine martial artist, may have probed and learned the fighting system quickly from these assertive women. In turn, she trained Yim Wing Chun, who was also inspired by the attitude of these powerful women. What Abbess Ng Mui and Yim Wing Chun learned from these women was probably some fighting methodology based on both the female structure and female thinking. Later, Yim Wing Chun and her husband probably systematized it to the point where their descendants were able to develop it further to the concise and compact system we now have today.

Nowhere in the history of the martial arts did any woman make a name for herself as much as Abbess Ng Mui and Yim Wing Chun. Martial arts have always been traditionally dominated by men; the fact that Wing Chun differs so much from other traditional Chinese martial arts tells me that men didn't create it.

The Yijikim Yeungma stance of Wing Chun is another big clue to the art's feminine origins. The knee-in leg position simply isn't a "manly" posture. Yijikim Yeungma (二字箝羊馬), translates to "Character Two Clamping Sheep Horse." It is a senseless phrase to non-Chinese and other martial artists. Remember, Chinese words and expressions are symbolic. In other words, they draw a picture in your mind. The number "2" in Chinese is depicted by a character representing two horizontal parallel lines, 二. So, what image would come to your mind when someone says "Two horizontal parallel lines clamping a sheep horse?" If you can't imagine, tell me what the symbol ;-) brings to your mind? Of course, we all know it because we use it commonly when typing with our keyboards. Because the keyboard does not have special characters that make up the winking face in the horizontal position, we get a tilted winking face instead. I remember the first time I saw the symbol and scratching my head to figure out what it meant. There isn't any Chinese character with two vertical parallel lines; however, the founders of Wing Chun had enough imagination to use existing Chinese characters to draw the picture they wanted to convey. So, if you tilt the 2 horizontal parallel lines to make it vertical, what do you get? *Two vertical parallel lines clamping the sheep horse.*

Got it? Well, I know you're now asking, "What the hell is a sheep horse?" In martial arts, the "horse" refers to your lower trunk. Chinese martial arts don't use the term "stance," because a stance denotes a static position. As the martial arts are related to (ancient) warfare, the horse better represents a person's lower trunk, legs, and movements. Now that we understand that, what does "Two vertical parallel lines squeezing the sheep stance" evoke in your mind? I'm sure New Zealanders and Australians would immediately see the picture. For those who can't, it is a picture of a person clamping the sheep's head between his thighs while shearing the wool.

Now, this is a significant clue that points the origin of Wing Chun to the Daliang Mountain in Southwest China instead of Henan, Fujian, Guangdong or anywhere in Southeast China—and here's why: Fujian Province (where the southern Shaolin Temple was located and where some claim Wing Chun originated), Guangdong Province (where Yim Wing Chun had lived), and the city of Foshan (where Dr. Leung Jan and Ip Man had lived) are all situated in the southeast coastal region of China, where the weather is classified as humid subtropical. Being at the coast, the main diet for the locals is seafood. The region is completely unsuitable for sheep grazing or breeding. There are no sheep to be found in southeast China, whereas, in northwest (in places like Inner Mongolia) and southwest China there are plenty of sheep for wool shearing and eating. Even in Henan, where the northern Shaolin Temple is located, sheep are not bred, sheared, or eaten. So, the expression Yijikim Yeungma couldn't have been coined in Fujian, Henan, or Guangdong. It wouldn't have invoked any sensible image to a Fujian or Guangdong practitioner, just as the winking icon wouldn't make sense to a Kalahari aborigine. It had to have been coined by people in the Daliang Mountain region, where wool shearing was a common sight, and such an expression would have made for an easy reference to a local activity.

In addition, I have observed through teaching Wing Chun over the decades that for most men, the difficult part of mastering Wing Chun is applying the concept of Yin (the counterpart of Yang). Yin represents femininity, softness, void and negativity, and is required to make the art whole. Men already possess plenty of Yang characteristics such as masculinity (testosterone/aggression), hardness (large muscles/forceful), substance (large bones/structure) and positivity (assertiveness/non-yielding). What they need is to cultivate their Yin qualities in order to neutralize and balance themselves, allowing them to become more holistic and more complete Wing Chun practitioners. Without the Yin characteristics, they are only half equipped. They will not be able to soften, avoid, and negate larger Yang forces than their own.

Denying the involvement of women in this art denies the Yin power within men. For this reason, men usually fail miserably in grasping the full concept of Wing Chun. The concept of Yin-Yang applied towards martial arts is not exclusive to Wing Chun; Tai Chi, Bagua, and other "soft" arts also make reference to Yin-Yang. However, who is to say that the other arts were not originally created by women (or by effeminate men), or that women at least had a hand in their creation, or that a woman's approach was at least brought into the development of these arts? Only men could be so arrogant as to deny the contributions of women to something so significant as martial arts. I understand that to many practitioners the history and origin of Wing Chun will not make a difference to their personal training or development. It is true that there is no concrete proof to back up the story of Abbess Ng Mui and Yim Wing Chun, but, by the same token, there exists no concrete proof to substantiate the other stories either. Great-Grandmaster Ip Man left us a great legacy by presenting us with the gift of Wing Chun Kuen. He showed gratitude and respect towards his master and those who came before him by naming each one of them right down to the art's originators. Many practitioners honor him by hanging a picture of him in their schools, but dismiss the involvement of the two matriarchs. I feel that those who receive the gift of Wing Chun and yet dismiss the Abbess Ng Mui and Yim Wing Chun are doing a great disservice to these women and are biting the hands that have fed them. They not only disrespect and dishonor the matriarchs but Great-Grandmaster Ip Man as well.

SIX

THE WING CHUN CONCEPT

WING CHUN IS A training program based on a concept of fighting as perceived by the founders of the art. Wing Chun is not a "style of fighting," because fighting, per se, has no style—and this is true of any martial art.

You can be a practitioner of Karate, Taekwondo, Jujitsu, Boxing, or Wing Chun, but your actions in a real fighting situation will not appear anything like they do in a sparring session with your fellow students. If you treat your martial art training program as a style and then attempt to always conform to it you will never be able to deal with even the most basic fighter in a real fight. Don't be fooled by watching the YouTube videos posted by instructors who make their moves and counter moves appear like something you would see in a well-choreographed Kung Fu film. When you see a video of an instructor taking apart three assailants who are posing as muggers, and doing so with cleanly choreographed and executed techniques, please realize that this is a show—it's not a real fight.

Any martial art that you care to name is just a fighting concept; a concept developed by the art's founder. The concept may be to make yourself a moving and difficult target to hit, or to stay grounded and use a gate-system for defense, or condition yourself to take the hardest blows, or to deliver your strikes from a certain "ideal" distance, or to be an inside or close-range fighter, or to immobilize an opponent by locking up his joints, or slamming him to the ground, or all of the above. Whatever the concept, there then needs to be a training program that will provide the practitioner with the mental and physical conditioning required to understand and implement the concept in a combative situation.

Before we proceed, we should first define our terms. The dictionary states that a concept is "an idea or mental picture of a group or class of objects formed by combining all of their aspects." I think I can describe it in simpler terms by saying that "a concept is a set of ideas or principles that fit together in a non-contradictory manner to form a holistic whole."

This dictionary also describes training as "the action of teaching a person or animal a particular skill or type of behavior." It describes a program "as (1) a set of related measures, events, or activities with a long-term aim, (2) arrange according to a plan or schedule, (3) a series of coded software instructions to control the operation of a computer or other machine, (4) cause a person or animal to behave in a predetermined way."

In teaching martial arts, I have no interest in the fourth definition that describes programming as a method of causing a person "to behave in a predetermined way." This definition may very well apply to animals, computers and machinery, but certainly not to human beings. Unfortunately, this is exactly how a lot of teachers from various martial arts schools train their students. I am, however, deeply interested in training my students to be able to think and act for themselves. I like definition Number 3, but it requires some editing for martial arts application. I would reword it to read as, "a series of instructions to assist the trainee in controlling both his actions and those of his opponent."

The reason why I have no interest in causing a person to behave in a predetermined way is that no one can predict how an opponent will attack. This approach also leads one down the path of being an accumulator of techniques for the sake of accumulating techniques—as if the more techniques one collects, the safer one will be in a fight. Again, the dictionary reveals that a technique is "(1) a way of carrying out a task, especially the execution or performance of an artistic work or a scientific procedure, (2) a skillful and efficient way of doing or achieving something." I like both descriptions very much, however this is not how most martial artists view the definition of technique. They believe a technique to be the perfect predetermined reaction to a specific action. In other words, if your opponent throws a punch in a certain way, then you must respond in a certain manner with a certain block and/or strike; e.g., if your opponent throws a roundhouse kick at you, then you must use a double-arm block, etc. To me a technique is more about body alignment and leverage and how I execute a particular movement in a skillful and efficient manner.

For example, when doing the Tansau movement in Wing Chun (one of the movements revealed in the Siu Nim Tau form), the correct technique would ensure that my palm and fingers are both fully stretched but in a relaxed manner, with my wrist in a slightly extended position, my elbow aligned to my middle fingertip, my upper arm and forearm in the same vertical plane and my radial bone in contact with the inside of my opponent's arm. I would feel the radius contact on the heel of my predominant leg, I would have my upper torso connected with my lower trunk, I would feel the force traveling toward my opponent's Centerline, etc. What I do with my other limbs and body parts would then depend upon the situation at every moment that unfolds thereafter, but each movement would be executed with the same precision that the Tansau was designed for; and not simply from a predetermined set of actions that I learned in a martial arts class. In other words, I would make that decision instantly, and tweak my Tansau and other body parts to fit the situation instead of taking a snap shot of the situation, and then attempting to match it with the scenario that I practiced in class.

If you rely on predetermined scenario techniques, you will never be able to amass enough of them. If you prepare for ground fighting, you may end up fighting standing up, or in the water, in the snow, or on the edge of a hill. If you prepare solely for knife fighting, you may end up facing a guy with a baseball bat instead. So, what is the solution? The solution is to train in a universal system that has a good overall fighting concept that will prepare your mind and nervous system to deal with most, if not all, types of situations.

The legendary samurai Musashi Miyamoto who survived sixty real life-and-death duels, and without much formal training, met all of his challengers unprepared, and, armed with just a stick or a wooden sword, often killed experienced samurais who were armed with razor sharp swords and spears. When he grew older he retired to live in a cave and contemplate Zen. There he wrote a book entitled *The Book of Five Rings*. This book had little to do with physical martial arts techniques or the weapons that he used in his numerous battles. Instead it was about his thoughts on fighting—his concepts, strategy and mindset. It was this mindset, Musashi believed, that was responsible for his success in battle.

The last section of his book is entitled *The Book of Void* and this is the shortest of all of the sections in his book and is also the most important. It deals solely with the spirit, something very, very few martial artists understand or connect with during the course of their careers. Only the best of them ever make this connection. When you can bring your mind to a void, everything becomes crystal clear. In essence, you can make time stand still or slow it down. When you enter into a fight with an empty mind, that is to say, without any preconceived or predetermined ideas, then you are capable of making quick decisions and adaptations based upon the pulse of the moment without any deliberation, encumbrance from thoughts, feelings, or desires. The attainment of the void mindset is the highest level of martial art.

Similarly, in Chinese history the Chinese military general Sun Tzu wrote the acclaimed book *The Art of War* sometime between the third and sixth century BCE. *The Art of War* is generally considered to be the first book ever published on the science of warfare and is still studied by military and business schools worldwide. As with Musashi, Sun Tzu did not deal with the use of particular weapons or military techniques, but rather with how to direct the mind during battle. He noted that:

"In battle, there are no more than two methods of attack—direct and indirect; yet these two will give rise to endless series and combinations of maneuvers."

Sun Tzu understood that what is most important is not a matter of knowing a lot of techniques, but rather of knowing the principles or concepts of efficient warfare. Once one understands these principles and concepts, the techniques will arise spontaneously as the situation requires.

In other words, once you understand the concept of fighting, per se, and attain the proper mindset, you will be able to make the correct decisions and maneuvers during a fight without any deliberation. Your mind will have the ability to change its focus from super-macro to super-micro in an instant, and vice versa; your vision will catch the slowest to the fastest movements; your actions will be precise and sharp. When you reach this level, it doesn't matter what tools you use for the same reason that for an imaginative and skilled photographer, it doesn't matter what camera he has in his hands, he will always take fantastic pictures. This is the reason people such as Muhammad Ali, Bruce Lee, David Beckham, Sidney Crosby, and others like them have stood out above their peers in each of their respective fields. The rules (in the case of sports) and the tools they used in developing their skills weren't all that different than those used by their peers, however these people excelled far beyond them. Did they possess any particular recognizable technique that can be attributed to their respective successes that you could adopt to use successfully? No, I don't believe they did. Did they have a style? Yes, but only their own. For each of them, their special ability, like Musashi, was their mindset. Their ability to understand the game on a higher level than the others and to be able to adapt instantly to any changes they encountered from moment to moment. They each possessed an ability to make opportunities happen instead of waiting for them to arise. Those who train and wait for the ideal situation to arise will never see it occur. This is why it is important to have an empty mind that is able to process events as quickly as they unfold without any distraction or deliberation—and this is why Wing Chun is such a fantastic combative concept with an equally as fantastic training program.

Many sifus describe Wing Chun as a form of close-quarter fighting, or that it is about cultivating fast hands, rapid footwork, powerful strikes, soft defense, adept mobility and other such things. However, they have missed the forest for the trees. What they are describing are merely properties or attributes that flow forth from the concept, what Bruce Lee called "segments of the totality" of fighting. The concept that gives birth to these attributes is where the real gold from Wing Chun (or any other martial art) is to be found.

So, what is Wing Chun's concept of fighting and training method? There are many components that make up the Wing Chun concept. If I were to attempt to wrap them all up in a simple one-line answer, it would be, "whatever it takes to neutralize the situation in the safest, most efficient, effective, and economical manner as possible." That's the bottom line when it comes to dealing with a conflict. In a physical fight, you'd knee, choke, head-butt or bite your opponent if that is what it would take to neutralize him in the safest, most efficient, effective, and economical way. The fact that head-butting or biting is not in any of the Wing Chun forms doesn't mean that you cannot use these options when necessary or when the opportunity arises. They're not in the training curriculum because they're natural instinctive survival tools for humans, which don't require particular attention or training. By contrast, there is much to develop when it comes to rooting oneself to the ground, unifying different units of the body, or throwing a powerful punch.

Similarly, there are many components to Wing Chun's training method, so to attempt to wrap them all up in a simple one-line answer, it might be: "to raise the practitioner's consciousness to an extremely high level." When a person's consciousness is extremely acute, he becomes aware not only of all of his own actions, but also his opponent's actions, as well as the activities that are going on around him. In essence, the mechanism in his brain begins firing at a faster rate than normal. At such a rate, other people's actions will become slow to him, or, conversely, his actions will become faster than theirs. This higher level of conscious awareness will allow him to be able to read a situation sooner and more accurately than he would normally. He will see or sense a glass toppling off a table before others do, and, therefore, he will be able to react sooner than others would in catching it. To other people, he will appear to have quicker reflexes than them. However, in actuality, it is his acute conscious awareness that allows him to read the situation sooner, and, therefore, to act sooner. All good athletes have developed this ability, whether it is Ali, Gretzky, or Beckham. Thus, the ultimate goal of Wing Chun training is to raise the consciousness of the trainee. He will learn to sense the inner workings of his physical body and mind. He will learn to sense his opponent's actions and thoughts. Ultimately he will perhaps sense the workings of the universe. It is only when he is fully aware of his own body and mind, of other people's bodies and minds, and of his surroundings, that he can then exercise some control over these things.

SEVEN

WING CHUN AND *THE ART OF WAR*

THE WORD "MARTIAL" REFERS to anything military. "Art" refers to the human expressions of creativity, skill, beauty and culture. Another moniker for martial art is "the art of war" or "the science of warfare." Wing Chun's concept of fighting is based on the concept of warfare in the large, rather than just a microscopic aspect of this concept, such as two people fighting each other.

To the Wing Chun practitioner, the human body is regarded as a fort or a mobile camp. The head is the most important component of the fort because that is where the commander (your brain) resides. The commander issues orders from the top of the fort or hill where he has a good overview of the battlefield. The body's Centerline can be likened to the stairway that leads to the commander, his lines of communication, and his chief officers. The Centerline Plane, the plane that connects one body Centerline to another, is the path leading to both the fort and its commander. All attacks should be focused on them. They should be attacked directly from the front, side, outside, inside, top and bottom simultaneously. In order to do this effectively, the commander sends out his spies to learn anything and everything they can about the enemy's commander. During a fight your main objective is to capture, immobilize, maim, or destroy the enemy commander, thus cutting off all communication from him to his officers and soldiers. His army will be nothing without him.

In order to have a strong defense the fort must be stable and strong. It should be designed with a moat around it as its inner line of defense to keep away or slow down the enemy's troops from penetrating the fort's main gate. Guards should be assigned to protect the east and west wings, as well as the ground, middle and top floors of the fort. The top floor, where the commander resides, takes top priority. Guards assigned for the east and west wings are given specific instructions not to leave their posts unless the other wing is compromised, and then to return quickly to their posts when the compromised wing is secured again.

An army that is properly prepared for battle should consist of an offensive team and a defensive team. In a battle, to occupy or destroy the enemy's fort, the offensive team should focus on penetrating the fort and destroying the commander and his officers. The defensive team should assist the offensive team by diverting any and all attacks coming at them from the enemy's offensive team. It should also constantly provide information to its commander regarding the enemy's movements and present status.

In a battlefield where camps are set up, the horsemen are trained to advance and to keep up the pressure on the enemy's soldiers. If the enemy starts to overwhelm them they should not retreat unless absolutely necessary. If necessary, they must fortify a new camp and fight to regain the lost ground. The objective is to continue pressing on until the enemy has retreated or has been immobilized or defeated.

In Wing Chun's warfare strategy, the body parts assume the roles of the fort, camp, moat, gates, commander, guards, weapons, and defensive and offensive teams. Because of the numerous roles required, the body parts play and change roles as often as necessary. For example, the three sections of the arms are given three roles to play. The hands take the role of offense, the forearms take the role of defense, and the upper arms take the role of fortification. However, each can switch roles as required so long as doing so allows them to work more economically, efficiently, practically and productively. The hands take the role of the offensive team, as they are the furthest from our body but the closest to the body of our opponent. The forearms take the role of the defensive team, as they're right behind the offensive team, as well as in front of the fortifying upper arms. The upper arms take the role of fortification because they are closest to the body (the fort). They play the role of guards that prevent enemy entry should the enemy penetrate the defensive team.

Many fighting systems use the hands (particularly the palms) for defense or fortification. Once the hands are used for this, however, they cannot be used as a weapon again without first disengaging from their role as defender. Thus, most martial arts segregate defense and offense as two separate and distinct actions. However, if the hand is used for attacking, and the forearm or upper arm is used to deflect or stop the opponent's attack simultaneously, then the whole process is narrowed down to but a single action, which makes the process much more economical, efficient and productive.

THE CHINESE CONNECTION—REDUX

Chinese culture and history is very much intertwined. Every aspect of Chinese life is influenced or based on historical events and people. Whether it was the first or last emperor, Qin or Qing Dynasty, Confucius or Laozi, Sun Tzu or Yuefei, Chinese medicine or inventions, they have all influenced the political, religious, martial, and family structures of China. Wing Chun is made up of all of these factors as well. Make no mistake, Wing Chun is a product of Chinese culture. Without having knowledge and experience of Chinese culture and history, the Wing Chun practitioner will only skim over the surface of his art. But the Wing Chun practitioner who takes the time to understand Wing Chun holistically will come to see the *Tao Te Ch'ing*, *The Art of War*, Traditional Chinese Medicine, and Confucianism within it. Wing Chun borrows and implements the philosophy of Yin-Yang from Taoism, the mindset from *The Art of War*, Qi and the meridians from Traditional Chinese Medicine, and the hierarchal family system from Confucianism. Many of the Wing Chun Kuit (訣, secret sayings) were drawn from these sources.

It is very important to understand what the founders of Wing Chun had in mind in terms of the strategy necessary to overcome an opponent. The Wing Chun strategy was never so much about tactical maneuvers, but rather about equipping the trainee with the mental, physical, emotional and spiritual means to deal with the unexpected, the unknown and the unpredictable. General Sun Tzu had already written a treatise on the strategies of warfare in *The Art of War*. Everything one needed to know about warfare was summarized within its thirteen chapters. As a result, it wasn't necessary for the Wing Chun founders to write another book on the strategies of martial action. They just needed to ensure that the training program they designed adhered to the valid philosophy and strategies expressed in that book. All that the Wing Chun founders needed to do was to complement the insights of the book with a training program for the practitioner of their art. While Sun Tzu's book covered the mental understanding of warfare, the training program would need to lay the groundwork to prepare the trainee physically, emotionally, and spiritually for such understanding. Sun Tzu cleverly strategized warfare in such a way that it could be studied and used in any era against any type of opponent. The thirteen chapters of *The Art of War* are as follows:

1. Assessment and Planning
2. Economics of War

3. Strategic Attack
4. Tactical Positioning
5. Directing Forces
6. Weak and Strong Points
7. Maneuvers
8. Variations and Adaptability
9. Movement and Development of Troops
10. Environment
11. Nine Situations
12. Fiery Attack
13. Intelligence and Espionage

The following is an overview of the first seven chapters of *The Art of War*, and how closely the principles of Wing Chun align with those contained within Sun Tzu's treatise.

ASSESSMENT AND PLANNING

The first thing that Sun Tzu said about assessment and planning is that, "The art of war is of vital importance to the State." I can't recollect any wars in human history that weren't fought over the occupation or defense of a territory (state), property, or way of life. In the Wing Chun System, our body is the property or the castle we are defending. The ground that the castle occupies is our territory. Sun Tzu said, "The art of war is a matter of life and death, a road either to safety or ruin." Similarly, the Wing Chun System is designed to protect your castle, property, and life. "The art of war is governed by (1) the moral law, (2) heaven, (3) earth, (4) commander, (5) method and discipline." In Wing Chun, the moral law is the principle that governs Wing Chun. The heaven signifies the heavenly environments (weather) that affect the warfare. The earth signifies the earthly environment (terrain) that affects the warfare. The commander is the brain that commands the body for action and courage. The method and discipline correlate to the Wing Chun training system and forms. Here are some other main quotes from Sun Tzu in Chapter One:

> According to conditions, we must modify our plans.
> All warfare is based on deception. Therefore, when we are able to attack, we must appear unable; when using our forces, we must appear idle; when we are close, we must make the enemy believe we are distant; when distant, we must make him believe we are close.
> Set baits to entice the enemy. Fake disorder, and destroy him.

If he is fully secured, be prepared for him. If he is stronger, avoid him. If he is lax, don't give him rest. If his forces are united, break them up.

Attack where he is unprotected; attack where he least expects.

Do not divulge your military plans or weaponry beforehand.

Most Wing Chun practitioners move about much more than is necessary when sparring. Subconsciously, they emulate and perform like actors they've seen in action movies. In the movies, the protagonist will move from one end of the room to another; from one room to another; from one building to another; he will perform a lot of blocking with his arms clashing repeatedly with those of his opponent before making his big surge to win the fight. If you understand warfare, it's about standing one's ground, holding the fort, breaking through the enemy's castle and occupying its territory. Therefore, when the enemy directs its force towards your castle and territory, you don't move the castle, territory and your army out of the way. You hold your ground and fight them off. In addition, you attack not only to dispel them, but to occupy their territory. The objective for both armies is to break through the castle's gate, enter the castle and capture and destroy the commander. One never retreats unless one is being overpowered. You don't penetrate the gates of a castle and then withdraw, and then look to repeat the whole process over and over. You must continue to press on until you've overpowered your enemy. I see Wing Chun practitioners retreating every time the opponent attempts an attack. Not only that, they block the attacks while in retreat—in effect performing a double defense. The fact is that if you back up, you've already put yourself out of harm's way, so there exists no need to use your arm to block the attack. Doing so simply means you've invested energy into a move that was superfluous, which doesn't equate to efficiency, which is the touchstone of the art of Wing Chun. It should be pointed out that whenever you step back out of harm's way, you've also moved your opponent out of harm's way. If he can't hit you, then you can't hit him either—unless, of course, you have a tremendous reach advantage over him. Even this would be less productive because when a body is moving backward, the forward projected punch is not as powerful as it is when thrown from a stationary position or thrown in conjunction with a body that is moving forward. The concept of Wing Chun is to make defense and offense one indivisible whole, just as Yin-Yang represents two components that make up one indivisible whole. So, the purest Wing-Chun way of dealing with an attack is to stay grounded and fire off a defensive and an offensive hand simultaneously (or, better still, fire off an offensive foot in your opponent's direction as well).

I see this retreating problem creeping into Wing Chun as a result of the way many students (and not a few teachers of the art) practice their Chisau (黐手, Sticking Hands—an exercise unique to Wing Chun) training these days. When one person attempts an attack, and the other always retreats. They look like they're dancing around a ballroom! There is no sense of one protecting one's territory at all. In the battleground, you don't retreat every time your enemy marches or charges forward; you hold your ground and fight them off. In fact, your commander not only expects you to hold your ground, but commands his troops to charge at their enemy to gain ground. He will only call for his army to retreat when he sees that it is being overpowered.

The problem with most Wing Chun practitioners today is that they are not training to strengthen their structure and balance. Thus, they're not confident enough to hold their ground, or perhaps they are unable to do so because of not developing strength in their structure and balance. Many practitioners talk about structure these days, but I haven't seen many that know what it entails. Your body must have a strong structure like a castle and you cannot have a strong castle if it is erected on a weak foundation.

The first form of Wing Chun, Siu Nim Tau (小念頭, literally translated as Little Reading Head), can be considered a user's manual for the novice, as it contains the fundamentals of the Wing Chun system. Without these fundamentals, there is no foundation to build upon. Siu Nim Tau introduces and teaches you the principles of Wing Chun, the nature of human anatomy, the laws of physics and how they all work together harmoniously. It introduces the practitioner to the main hand tools of the art of Wing Chun and how to use them. It teaches you to root your structure deeply to the ground (like the foundation of a castle), how to amalgamate different parts of your body into one unit (like a solidly-built castle) and, when necessary, to isolate and detach single units—and also how to synchronize your mechanical gears (muscles and joints) and levers (bones) to deliver maximum impact force while employing minimum effort. I believe that the Wing Chun founders based their training program on Sun Tzu's thesis, designing the Siu Nim Tau form to provide the trainee with a strong structure, good balance and powerful weapons. I believe that they designed the Chum Kiu form (the second form of Wing Chun) to provide the trainee with a strong and unfaltering warhorse. And that they designed Biu Jee (the third empty-hand form of Wing Chun) to provide the trainee with an extraordinary arsenal of weapons and skills.

Wing Chun training does not prepare the practitioner for specific combative situations or environments because these can be endless. Every opponent, situation or environment will be different from the one that you practiced training for at your Wing Chun school. Every sparring occurrence or fight will be different from the previous one, just as every chess, football or hockey game will occur differently from previous ones. You just cannot replicate it. To think that a fight will go down exactly in the manner that you had trained for it, or that you will know ahead of time what your opponent will do, is simply wishful and unrealistic thinking. Sun Tzu, Musashi, and the founders of Wing Chun knew this very well, with the result that they never instructed their students on any preset maneuvers. They just provided the necessary concepts that could be used and made to fit in with any given situation and environment.

Sun Tzu said:

Don't repeat tactics that have gained you one victory, but let your methods be determined by the infinite variety of circumstances. Just as water retains no constant shape, there are no constant conditions in warfare. He who can modify his tactics in relation to his opponent can be called a natural-born leader.

Musashi said:

The true value of sword fencing is not within the confines of sword-fencing techniques.

Wing Chun's concept regarding circumstantial and environmental fighting is this: You should be able to fight anyone, anytime, and anywhere, as long as you know how the human body and the physical laws of the universe work, and how to make them work for you. After all, it is a man you will be fighting—whether you are on solid ground, sand, snow, in the water or in the sky, whether you are standing, sitting, or lying down. The laws of physics apply in each situation and environment. If you possess more knowledge of biomechanics and the laws of physics than your opponent, and if you have trained in a well-engineered system, then the likelihood of your overcoming your opponent is optimized.

THE ECONOMICS OF WAR

Sun Tzu understood the cost of war, and that victory most often goes to the commander who best manages the economics of wealth, production, and consumption. In the combative arts, the management of economics does not mean running a gym or selling uniforms and other products to students. Economics in martial arts mean the management of mind, energy, and body. In the Chinese language, there are three very similar sounding words: *Yi, Qi* (pronounced *chee),* and *Li,* and it is important that they be clearly understood.

Yi (意) means "intention," Qi (氣) means "energy," and Li (力) means "physical strength."

Note that Qi does not actually translate to energy. The literal translation is "air." The ancient Chinese doctors and scientists used the word *air* to represent all that are in the air, such as electrons, protons, neutrons, photons, gases, bacteria, particles, etcetera, that they couldn't determine at the time. However, they did know that there were components in the air that affected living matters. For one, it energized living beings. To delve into the topic of Qi would take volumes of books to clarify; therefore, for the sake of simplicity, I will just describe Qi as energy, as many other writers have done.

A good martial artist must know how to manage all three of these attributes as economically as possible. An action must begin with Yi (intent), followed closely by Qi (energy) and end with Li (physical action). If you think about it, you'll recognize that we do this daily with all of our actions but for most actions it's not a linear, conscious process but rather a process that is performed subconsciously, particularly as we become more proficient at the things we do. For example, we have no problems running down a flight of stairs or playing a familiar musical instrument; however, when we are first introduced to a new task, we are now called upon to manage these three components consciously. When we run down a flight of stairs, we begin with the intent (Yi); i.e., we subconsciously say to ourselves that we "need to make it down to the main floor." At this point, the mind (Yi) automatically generates the energy (Qi) necessary to activate the nerves to engage the necessary muscles (Li) required to move your leg for the first step. Once the first step is taken, Yi quickly repeats the process for the second step without your having to consciously plan for it. The process is quick but synchronized, in a manner that has the Li running just ahead of the Qi, and the Qi running just ahead of the Li. Suppose your Yi (intent) was too strong and ran ahead of the Qi (energy); the Qi would need to suddenly sprint forward to catch up with Yi, and the Li (muscles/physical action) would be over-fueled to catch up with the Yi and Qi, resulting in the Li running ahead of Yi and Qi, causing them to move out of sequence and, thus, your control; then, your body would land on the ground sooner than intended. If your intent is too strong when learning to play the piano, for example, you will over-fuel your muscles with Qi; your fingers will stiffen and they will bang on the piano keys harder than is required; they would, in effect, be running ahead of Yi and you would end up depressing the wrong keys. When you are relaxed, your intent runs just ahead of the Qi, which runs just ahead of the Li to fuel the fingers you had intended to move. The process repeats for each finger action. In martial arts, when your Yi (intent) is too strong for an action, your facial expression and body language change and telegraph your intent to your opponent. Not only that, but you will over fuel your muscles, and your action will outpace your intent. When you are over-focused (too much Yi) on one action, you will not be aware of your opponent's actions or his changes in position, and, thus, you will not be able to adapt quick enough. When you do not manage your Yi, you will lose control of your Qi and Li. When you overuse your Qi, you will run out of fuel, and your Li will become impaired.

STRATEGIC ATTACKS

Sun Tzu believed in breaking the enemy's resistance without fighting. In the words of Bruce Lee, "Fighting without fighting," or "Winning without Fighting." A Wing Chun practitioner should always have the attitude that he can resolve a conflict without ever having to resort to fighting. Indeed, if he's clever enough, a good Wing Chun practitioner can walk away with a win-win situation without any punches being thrown. Sun Tzu said:

> The topmost generalship is derailing the enemy's plans; the next best strategy is preventing the conjunction of enemy's forces; next in line is attacking the enemy in open terrain; and the worst is attacking fortified cities; they are too costly and problematic.

As a Wing Chun fighter, you must thwart your opponent's every move by attacking him before or as he attacks you. You must not block, retreat or shift to put yourself in a defending or retreating position. Instead, you must prevent your opponent from combining his forces against you; you must conjunct your various forces against his singular force. You must attack the opponent where he is vulnerable, or work to create an opening for such an attack. You must take the fight outside of your own castle gates and inside your opponent's gates. You must create strong walls and gates to thoroughly secure your castle, thus making it costly and difficult for your opponent to penetrate. Conversely, you must enter via your opponent's walls and gates that are unsecured rather than attempting to break through ones that are well fortified.
Sun Tzu:

> "The commander who is impatient will launch his men to assault like swarming ants, with the result of one-third of his men being slain, while the town still remains untaken."

Far too often I have seen a Wing Chun practitioner charge at his opponent with a barrage of "chain punches," even though his opponent is well protected and out of striking range. Such attacks are initiated without a target, focus, or aim. The action is just a classic case of impatience combined with poor tactics and zero strategy. Sun Tzu cleverly advised: "If you and your enemy are equally matched, go into a battle; if you are a little inferior, avoid the battle; if you are quite disproportionate, take flight."

In Wing Chun, when you pair up with your opponent, your first priority is to stand your ground and overpower him. When he makes the first move, and you make contact, you will then find out where his strengths and weaknesses lie. Remember that even if he is larger than you, his structure may be weak (i.e., his body units are not united), and this will provide you with the opportunity to attack (and possibly destroy) his structure and unbalance him. If he is larger than you and his body units are semi-united, you can steer away or diffuse his force, and counter-attack when you have control of him. If he is larger than you and his body units are unified, and you are unable to break, unbalance or diffuse his force, you should retreat to the next ground (take one step to the side or back), which will allow you to regroup your units for new stratagems. This type of reaction or response aligns with Sun Tzu:

> If you know the enemy and yourself, you can go into a hundred battles without fear. If you know yourself but not the enemy, you will suffer defeat for every victory gained. If you know neither the enemy nor yourself, you will succumb to every battle.

TACTICAL POSITIONING

In an episode of the television series *Longstreet*, Bruce Lee's character is shown coming to the aid of a blind private detective who has been set upon by three thugs. After dispatching his adversaries, Lee is asked by the blind man, "What did you do to them?" His answer, for those who know the art, comes right out of Wing Chun: "They did it to themselves." According to Sun Tzu,

"It is within our own hands to secure ourselves against defeat; however, the opportunity to defeat the enemy is provided by the enemy himself." Hence a skillful fighter puts himself into a position that makes him invincible and does not miss any opportunity of defeating his opponent."

In Wing Chun training, we are made aware of our Centerline (our vulnerabilities), and how to protect it. By the same token, we understand the enemy's vulnerabilities and securities. Securing our commander and castle is of the utmost priority. When the enemy gives us a target to hit, we hit it. It's that simple. The enemy always provides the opportunity (or opportunities) necessary to defeat him. As Sun Tzu said, "In military methodology, you must first have assessment, estimation, and calculation to weigh the chances of victory." The Chisau exercise and the balance-and-structure exercises that I include in my classes teach my students to measure the opponent at first contact, estimate the quantity of his strength, make calculations regarding his force relative to theirs, their ability to neutralize (or balance) his force against theirs; and finally, the opportunity to use all of these factors to achieve victory.

DIRECTING FORCE

Sun Tzu wrote that "Controlling a large force is the same as controlling a small force; it's only a question of dividing up the numbers."

To ensure that your force is able to withstand the pressure of the enemy's attack and remain unbroken, you must implement direct and indirect maneuvers.

In all battles, the direct method is used for joining a battle; however, it is the indirect methods that will secure victory.

Indirect tactics are limitless and unending as the flow of rivers; and, as the sun and moon, they will end but always begin anew. Like the four seasons, they pass but will always return.

In battles, there are just two methods of attack—direct and indirect; yet the combinations of the two mutate and multiply to endless maneuvers.

The direct and indirect methods take turns leading each other. It is like walking in circles—you never come to an end.

Be deceitful in appearance, and keep the enemy on the move. Bait the enemy into a trap by making small sacrifices.

A skilled commander combines forces; he doesn't put demands on individuals. He is able to choose the right men and use combined energy.

When he combines energy, his men become rolling rocks. It is the nature of a rock to remain still on level ground, and move on a slope. When it is square, it stands still; when it is round, it rolls down.

Wing Chun's training program teaches you to utilize direct and indirect force, individually and cooperatively. You treat all of your bones, joints and muscles as gears or lever systems. The muscles and the energy that power the movement of bones and joints are always considered as force or effort. The bone shafts are used as levers, whereas the bone ends are often used as

[61]

fulcrums. Your heels and/or your whole structure standing on the ground provide the ultimate fulcrum. The joints are used to combine two or more lever forces. Each section of the lever system can be used individually or cooperatively with others. You can use these levers individually to conserve energy, and/or use them in combination to generate more power. Wing Chun forms, particularly the Siu Nim Tau form, teaches the practitioner this as it reveals the different tools of Wing Chun and how to use them individually (isolated movements) and cooperatively (synchronized movements). Far too often, practitioners do not isolate their movements and only use combinational and out-of-sequence movements. This can be likened to sending three people to do a job that only requires one; and to makes matters worse, if the three people have not coordinated their tasks it will result in a botched up job. Such an assignment becomes not only a waste of manpower, but a waste of money and is highly counter-productive. However, if three people with different skills and responsibilities took three parts of the job, and worked simultaneously in a well-coordinated fashion they would finish the job three times sooner than one person operating by himself could, and the end result would be economical, efficient, and productive.

For example, although you have three parts to your arm—your hand, forearm and upper arm—you may wish to isolate and use just your wrist joint to lower your opponent's arm to create an opening for (or to deflect) an attack, instead of also lowering your forearm and upper arm. Using all three parts of the arm for this one defensive task would not be economical, efficient or effective. By using all three parts of your arm you will end up lowering both your forearm and your upper arm to both a position and angle that won't allow you to throw a powerful punch without first raising your forearm and upper arm to a higher plane. If, on the other hand, only your wrist was used to lower your opponent's arm, then your forearm and upper arm will still be aligned in an optimum position and angle to throw a powerful punch. Indeed, your punch could follow immediately after or even simultaneously with the drop of your wrist; making the three parts of your arm work separately yet congruently for an economical, efficient and highly effective result. In the first case, the three parts of the arm would not only be doing the same defensive job, but would require an additional two steps to occur in order to deliver your offensive action, thus, separating defense and offense as two distinctive actions; whereas in the second scenario, your wrist is assigned to do the initial defense, the upper arm is used to propel the forearm (which, during travel, will check your opponent's arm), and your hand is used to strike your opponent's body, making defense and offense one and the same, and allowing you to accomplish both tasks with one action, (or two at most).

In Wing Chun, one must learn to control ten segments of your body as easily as you can control one, and also control ten segments of your opponent's body with just one of yours. For example, if your opponent weighs 100 kilograms, and you weigh 70 kilograms, then he outweighs you by 30 kilograms or 43 percent (100/70). Because he has 43 percent more mass, according to the laws of physics if you try to resist his moving body force directly; i.e., having both of your shoulder points facing both of his shoulder points squarely (whereby your coronal plane is exactly parallel to his) and having your front Centerline Plane meet his directly (whereby both of you share the same median plane), you will simply be bulldozed over owing to the size differential. However, if you took a small angular step either forward or backward, and rotated your structure to have your coronal plane perpendicular to his, and your median (Centerline) plane running along his coronal plane, you will have, in essence, divided or cut his structure in half. In such a scenario, you will have use of both of your sagittal sides against your opponent's single side; you will have your Centerline Plane aimed at his body while his Centerline is not aimed at any part of yours. In this position, you will have all of your 70 kilograms available to you to attack him, while he will only have 50 kilograms available to him to resist you—suddenly the balance of force has swung to your favor. You now have a 20 kilograms or about 40 percent (70/50) advantage over him. When you bring your hands together to your Centerline Plane, you will merge the forces of your two sagittal sides. Then when you direct your bodily force to your hands against your opponent's side from this position, he will be the one who is bulldozed.

WEAK AND STRONG POINTS

You will succeed if you attack places that are unsecured. You can ensure defense if you hold on to positions that are secured. A commander is skillful when he attacks enemies that do not know what to defend; and is skillful in defending against enemies that do not know what to attack.

By knowing the enemy's disposition and concealing ours, we can keep our forces unified, and make the enemy's divided.

The enemy must not know where we intend to attack; he will then have to prepare against all possible attacks at many different locations; therefore, his forces will be spread thin in many directions; and the numbers we will face at any given location will be proportionately less.

Arouse the enemy to learn the principles of its actions and inactions. Force it to reveal itself in order for us to know its vulnerabilities.

Compare the enemy's army against yours to know where the strength is abundant and where it is deficient.

Hide your dispositions, so you will be safe from the most discreet spies and plots from the wisest commanders.

Do not repeat tactics that gave you one victory, but let the infinite variety of circumstances determine your actions.

Military tactics are like water; for water naturally runs from high places downwards.

Water shapes its course according to the ground it flows on; a soldier must work out his victory according to the opponent he encounters.

Water has no constant shape; neither does warfare have constant conditions.

—Sun Tzu

In Wing Chun, it is vital that you secure your Centerline, and attack your opponent's when it is not secured. It is quite natural for all fighters to want to attack the opponent's head and to defend their own; however, there is an array of vital points along a person's Centerline that most fighters ignore. Although Wing Chun practitioners are reminded over and over about attacking the Centerline, they often just go after their opponent's head even when it is well protected. By doing so, they are not only doing what is expected, but also revealing their dispositions. Focusing on just one point of attack—for example, the tip of the nose—is like attempting to punch a mosquito in flight. However, if you attack the Centerline core (the line running from the top of your opponent's head vertically down the center of his body), there are a multitude of targets to hit, making it much easier to land a strike. In other words, your target options have now become more visible, larger and slower.

When your arms make contact with those of your opponent, you must remain very soft and sensitive. When you engage with an opponent who is hard and insensitive, his energy will reveal his intentions, strengths and weaknesses, whereas yours will be concealed, thus enabling you to deceive and overpower him.

While Bruce Lee is the martial artist who popularized the saying "Be like water," as you can see from Sun Tzu, it is a very old Chinese combat philosophy. In a real-life fighting situation, your actions must be like water; flowing and adapting to your opponent's actions and the circumstances that he has created. The opposite of this is the martial artist who over focuses on a single action. He has a concept in his mind of needing to "explode" his power at the end of a strike, when, in actuality, all he will succeed in is contracting his opposing muscles at the end of that action. It is akin to flooring the gas pedal and then suddenly slamming the brakes on. Such an action has a distinctive beginning and an end. So with every end action, the need arises to start a new action. This certainly cannot be considered "flowing," can it? In order to make one action flow into the next, one should only contract the set of muscles required for the action and then immediately relax them so that they can be used again immediately or even switch to another set of muscles for another action. Eliminating the contraction of the opposing muscles at the end eliminates an extra step.

Many contemporary Wing Chun sifus pride themselves on creating three-step or four-step technical drills for their students. The danger inherent in this is that the student will then be programmed to respond mechanically rather than intuitively. The purpose of a drill is to repeat an action until it is ingrained in the practitioner's neural system; this way, the student needn't go through the slow process of "thinking" but rather lets his subconscious mind automate the desired action. However, if a student is drilled to respond in a certain way, and the opponent doesn't follow the sequence of the drill that the student has been practicing, then that student is out of luck. Anything more than one-step drills will fall into this trap; the practitioner's actions become a pattern of quickly predictable regularity; something Sun Tzu discouraged.

On the other hand, traditional one-step, non-sequential and highly intuitive drills, such as the Paksao Drill, has scores of variables that train the student in correct hand positioning, arm alignment, coordination, timing, judgment, sensitivity, the ability to discern or read force, control structure, balance, grounding, and footwork (among other attributes). It is more important to drill into the subconscious mind and neural system of the muscles the details and variables of a movement than to learn a combination of techniques. When you master each piece, it is very easy for the subconscious, intuitive, and instinctive mind to combine the various pieces you have learned and to quickly troubleshoot any unpredictable and unfamiliar problem.

MANEUVERS

An army without its supply train is lost; without provisions, it is lost; without a supply source, it is lost.

One cannot lead an army on the march without knowing the nature of the country—its mountains and forests, its caves and crevices, its marshes and swamps.

[65]

To merge or divide your troops must be determined by the circumstances.

Let your plans be dark as night, and move like lightning.

The way of retaining composure is to be disciplined and calm; look for disorder and confusion within the enemy.

Refrain from engaging an enemy who is orderly, calm, and confident.

It is a military rule to not advance uphill against the enemy, or to oppose him when he comes downhill.

—Sun Tzu

When fighting an opponent, you must conserve your energy and use it sparingly. You must know your opponent's disposition before engaging in a fight. You must assess the terrain or battleground and see how you can make it advantageous to you. You must maintain a calm demeanor so that your opponent is unable to read your disposition. Don't frown, cringe, or scowl because you cannot sustain such facial expressions during a fight. In order to unleash any attack quickly, you need to relax the opposing muscles of the ones required for the action you are initiating. Your subconscious already knows how to accomplish this (unless you've trained the movement to be consciously directed or your mind is so tense at the moment that it simply can't send the neural signal to the muscles without deliberation). When you strike, all of the muscles that are not required for the job should be relaxed—including your facial muscles. If the facial muscles are relaxed your opponent cannot read your face to be forewarned that a strike is about to come. By maintaining a calm disposition and expressionless face, your opponent will be in the dark. You must not change your expressionless face to a frown or scowl before, during, or after an action. First, it doesn't in any way speed up or power your actions; second, it will telegraph your actions; and third, it will just draw energy away from your working muscles to your face. Any muscle contraction requires energy to fuel it and fueling unnecessary muscle contraction is a waste of good energy.

Under each circumstance, you must know when to rest your body, when to use only a single body unit, and when to use more body units to deliver a thunderous attack. You must only use the amount of force required to get the job done—no more and no less. You must know when to borrow your opponent's force and when to use it to multiply your force against him. You must not resist his force directly; if he pushes your arm down, don't try to overpower him by pushing your arm back up. If he pushes your arm up, don't push your arm down directly against his force. Always direct his force *away* from its intended path and destination. Find the easiest and quickest

[66]

path to your opponent's Centerline. Don't look for resistance to overcome. When you detect the direction of your opponent's resistance (force), change your path of attack to one that encounters the least amount of resistance.

Don't attack your opponent blindly, especially when he is strongly guarded. If he is well guarded frontally, attack his side. If he is well guarded laterally, attack his front. If his upper zone is well guarded, attack his lower zone. If his lower zone is well guarded, attack his upper zone. If he appears to be strongly fortified generally, find his weakest fortification to break through.

In this chapter I've made comparisons between seven chapters of Sun Tzu's treatise *The Art of War* with Wing Chun's concepts on how to ensure victory over an opponent. You can do your own analyses with Sun Tzu's remaining six chapters, and I can assure you that you will find no contradictions between the two.

EIGHT

THE CENTERLINE: THE SCIENCE OF CONCENTRATION

THERE ARE MANY PRINCIPLES that flow forth from the Wing Chun concept like tributaries branching out from a mighty stream. One of these primary principles is that of the Centerline.

The Centerline is an imaginary line that runs vertically through the middle of one's body. In a broad sense, the Centerline principle can be found in almost every martial art. Even non-martial artists will instinctively punch or kick towards the center of an opponent's body. In this respect the action itself is not all that unique. However, when you probe deeper into the details of the principle as it is employed in Wing Chun, it becomes very unique.

Remember, Wing Chun is a fighting concept that has a group of ideas that adhere to a main theme, just like that of a country's constitution. The main principle and supreme law of The American Constitution reads:

We the people of the United States, in Order to form a more perfect Union, establish Justice, ensure domestic Tranquility, provide for the common defense, promote the general Welfare, and secure the Blessings of Liberty to ourselves and our Posterity, do ordain and establish this Constitution for the United States of America.

This supreme law derives the other laws of the United States of America. Wing Chun's supreme law, or at least its primary principle, is the Centerline. However, it is not just about defending your Centerline and attacking your opponent's Centerline. While attacking and defending the Centerline is the main goal, in order to achieve this goal specialized tools or weapons are required. However, in order to employ these tools, muscular power is required. And in order to effectively use muscular power, training is required. And in order to train properly, a system is required. And in order to implement the system, a strategy is required. And in order to implement a strategy, a goal is required. So, as you can see, a full circle is formed from mind (goal) to physical components (tools, muscular power, physical training), back to the mind again (mind training, strategy, and goal). From examining the list of components above, you can see that there are more mind components than there are physical ones. After all, physicality has limitations, whereas, the mind has none.

One's physical ability is limited by one's DNA, sex, environment, diet, and age. One's DNA is powerful; it determines how tall and how wide one will be. One's gender will also determine what kind of bones and muscles one will develop. One's environment and diet may allow one to fulfill one's physical capacity in terms of the ultimate size one may reach, but it will never be more than what one's DNA has already programmed the individual to develop. One's age will determine the ratio of cells that one's body will reproduce against how many will die off. This reproduction will continually drop off after a certain age, making one lose muscle mass (and the metabolic pathways within muscle) no matter how much one exercises.

I believe that the founders of Wing Chun took all of this into their calculus when formulating the principles of their art. They knew that at some point the Wing Chun trainee could expect to be placed at a physical disadvantage during a fight. After all, as the saying goes, "no matter how big or strong you are, there is always someone who is bigger and stronger"—and you may have to face this person one day.

This also lends more credence to the belief that Wing Chun is a martial art that was created by women; after all, which sex, on average, has to routinely overcome the greatest physical disadvantages in terms of size and strength? Without question it is the female sex. And if Ng Mui and Yim Wing Chun were not involved in the founding or development of Wing Chun, perhaps its male founders were on the slighter side and thus recognized that success in physical encounters against bigger and stronger males had to be predicated more on the female principle (Yin) than attempting to overcome a greater force directly with a lesser force. Recall that the Chinese opera troupes consisted solely of males and that those males who were slightest in physical stature were the ones selected to play the female roles in the operas. If such men were involved in the development of the art, then certainly they would have contributed their insights into this aspect of physicality.

The main principle behind the Centerline concept is focusing squarely on the goal of attacking your opponent's Centerline while simultaneously protecting our own. However, as simple as this may sound, it is not that easy to accomplish and requires focus. The reason why soccer superstar Renaldo was able to score as many goals as he did lay in his ability to focus on his objectives without being distracted from his goal by other players and/or spectators. The rules, tools, and training for the game of soccer are the same for everyone who plays it, and yet Renaldo was able to consistently score more often and was far more accurate with his kicks on net than were his peers. Was he just lucky enough to have the ball fall in front of him and to have an opportunity and opening to score? No, every player has the ball in front of him at some point and most get the chance to score, but they just don't do it as consistently as Renaldo did. Renaldo's mind was so focused on his objective that he saw opportunities that others simply didn't see. He had no particular techniques that were better than those employed by his peers; he simply experienced the game better than the others.

Similarly, it is vital that a Wing Chun practitioner understands the principle of the Centerline, and maintains that focus without distraction. The Centerline is not just a line drawn down the front surface of a person; it is actually a line running inside a person. Therefore, the focus point of one's attack and defense is also inside the person rather than merely the outer aspect. When you take this approach, it is easy to target the Centerline, whether your opponent is facing you from the front, the rear, from the side, or in any other position. You needn't create a different Centerline for every posture your opponent assumes. When you hit, you hit through your opponent to his center core, which will not only ensure that you reach your target but will also ensure that you deliver a more powerful strike in the process. Similarly, when you are defending, you are defending your inner core, rather than the outer surface. Because of this, you can even use the surface of your body as a defensive weapon.

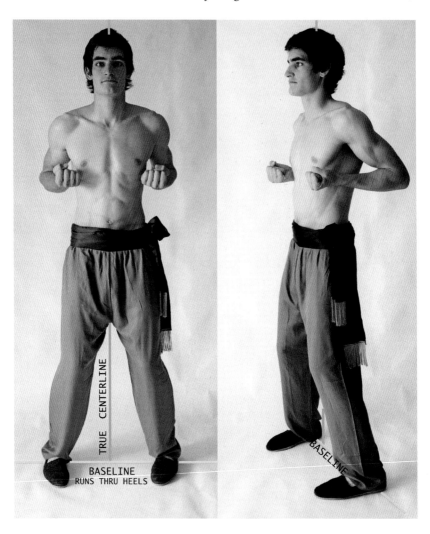

The true Centerline is a vertical line that runs perpendicular to the floor, from the pinnacle of the head, through the center of the body, and out of the perineum, down to the ground. One should attack the opponent's Centerline and protect one's own. Attacking the true Centerline will deliver a penetrating blow.

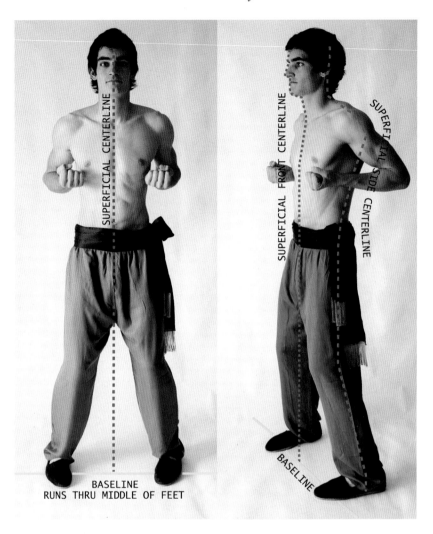

BASELINE
RUNS THRU MIDDLE OF FEET

Many Wing Chun practitioners mistakenly mark the Centerline on the surface of the body. Consequently, they are having to mark the sides and the back of the body for clarification. Whereas, the true Centerline, inside the body, is visible from all angles. Also, when the Centerline is marked on the surface of the body, one tends to focus on it as the target of attack. Unfortunately, it is only skin deep.

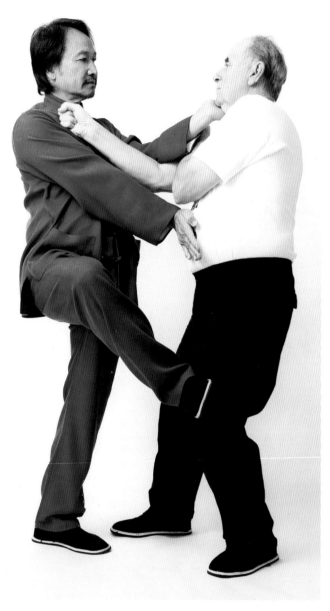

David punches Danny's Centerline. Rather than intercepting or deflecting David's punch with his arm(s), Danny uses his upper torso as a defensive tool to roll and diffuse the force of the punch by rotating it, thus freeing up both his arms, which he uses to attack David instead. When one is aware and protective of the true Centerline, he doesn't need to concern himself over the touch of the opponent's fist on the surface of the body. He can use the contact to read the opponent's force.

Besides the Centerline itself there is the Centerline Plane to be concerned with. This is the path that you will take to direct your offense, and the path that you will use to defend your center core. Having your weapons travel along this path will produce the most economical, efficient and productive result owing to the shortness and directness of the path of travel. Any contact you make with your opponent must be aligned and directed to your Centerline Plane if you're squared to your opponent, or to the heel of the rear and predominantly weighted leg if your structure is on an angle. This will ensure that your opponent's force will be well-resisted by your being firmly grounded (i.e., having your structure secured via your feet through your spinal column in a square position, or by your rear leg and one sagittal side when on an angle). By the same token, if the force coming at you is too strong to resist, then it can be dissolved by altering the alignment of your structure or your foot.

It is not uncommon for many Wing Chun practitioners to create many Gates and many Centerlines to further strengthen their positions. This is analogous to building a fort with many different gates and stairways. Unfortunately, creating so many Gates (entryways and guards) and Centerlines (paths and stairways) require more finance, more manpower, and more management. Also, the more entryways and paths you create, the more openings are available to your opponent to enter and attack your fort. Not only will your economy and manpower be unmanageable and spread too thin, but it will give a centralized enemy even more power and opportunity to penetrate your defense.

THE WING CHUN FORT

In reality, the Wing Chun "fort" has but one vertical plane that is divided into three horizontal planes. The vertical plane is the median body plane that divides the left and right sagittal planes. In Wing Chun, it is called the Centerline Plane. The Centerline Plane on the body originates from the center of the body but is also the line of gravity that runs through the body. It runs from the pinnacle of the head through the center core of the body, and through the bottom region of the pubic area to the ground. When you view the vertical Centerline as a line running through the center core of the body instead of just its surface, you needn't have a front, side, oblique or back Centerline because the core line can be viewed and accessed from all angles. You can then protect your center core and attack your opponent's from every possible angle. When you treat the path from your center core to the opponent's as a Centerline Plane, then you needn't create any extra Centerlines between the cores. Instead, you simply protect each and every point on that plane on an equal basis. This should also be done at every point of the three horizontal planes within the body's structure as well. In other words, you simplify the fortification, defense and offense by setting up one vertical Centerline Plane to fortify, protect and attack, and three horizontal planes to fortify, protect, and attack.

A human being has but four limbs. To use these limbs for fortification and simultaneous defense and offense, at least one of your legs will need to be used for standing. You are then left with only three mobile limbs. Therefore, it is only logical to section the vertical plane into three horizontal planes so that each limb can then be used to protect these planes and also to attack your opponent. One arm can protect and attack the high region, from head to xiphisternum (xiphisternum plane), the other can protect and attack the middle zone, from xiphisternum to the spinous plane (where the spine meets the pelvis), while the free leg can protect and attack the lower zone, from the spinous plane to the foot on the ground. The design is simple yet effective. You use three limbs to defend your one Centerline Plane at three levels, and attack your opponent's Centerline along the Centerline Plane at three levels.

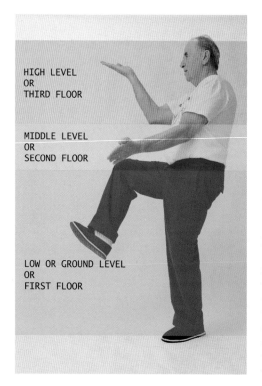

HIGH LEVEL
OR
THIRD FLOOR

MIDDLE LEVEL
OR
SECOND FLOOR

LOW OR GROUND LEVEL
OR
FIRST FLOOR

The Centerline is a vertical line running along the vertical core of one's body. The Centerline Plane is a vertical plane that aims and runs from one's Centerline to the opponent's Centerline. For the purpose of awareness and management, the Centerline Plane is divided into three horizontal levels, allowing three limbs to simultaneously attack the full length of the opponent's Centerline while defending one's own; or use the upper limbs singularly or dually to attack the opponent's Middle and High levels while defending one's own; or use the lower limbs to attack the opponent's Low level while protecting one's own.

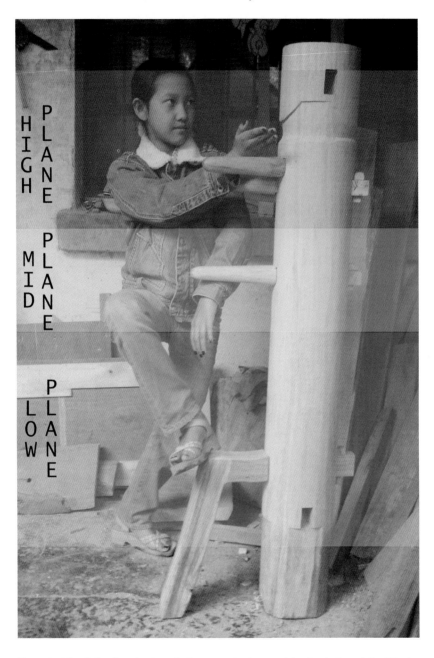

HIGH PLANE

MID PLANE

LOW PLANE

The principle of the three horizontal planes are implemented in the design of the Wooden Man, allowing the practitioner to use three limbs to simultaneously attack the opponent's Centerline Core, as well as defend own Centerline Core and Plane.

Both the concept and training method of Wing Chun were engineered to assist the Wing Chun practitioner in cultivating an indefatigable and unwavering focus upon his goal. That goal can be anything—from excelling in academics, to winning a game, to overpowering an opponent. Irrespective of the particular goal desired, in order to stay highly focused, the Wing Chun practitioner's focus must stay centered. In Chinese, the word for "center" is symbolized by a line cutting through a rectangular box (中). It is spelled *zhong* in Pinyin; pronounced *troong* in Mandarin and *cheong* in Cantonese.

In the vocabulary of Wing Chun, the words "Centerline" and "Centerline Plane" are often mistaken for one another, which can cause considerable confusion amongst practitioners of the art. In the Chinese language, these words are more distinctly demarcated: Centerline is represented by the characters 中心線, while Centerline Plane is represented by the characters 中線. (Although when you translate the term "Centerline" literally from English back to Chinese, it can be 中線; however, that's not how it is in the Chinese language or how it is represented in Wing Chun terminology). In English, "center" can be either a noun, verb, or an adjective, whereas in Chinese it can only be an adjective. In English, you can say, "He is in the center," or "That's the center." In Chinese, you can't finish these sentences with just the term for center (中), but must complete these sentences with a noun. To render such sentences into Chinese would leave them incomplete; prompting the questions: the "center of what?" Is it the "center point? The center line? The center of what objects?" In order to distinguish the difference between a person's Centerline and the Centerline Plane that projects from it, *Cheong Sam Sin* (中心線) or just *Cheong Sam* (中心) for short is used to represent the Centerline, and *Cheong Sin* (中線) is used to denote the Centerline Plane. In 中心, the word 中 (*cheong*) represents "center." The second character 心 (*Sam*) represents "heart." It also means "mind," "mindfulness," and "intent." It is pronounced *shin* in Mandarin and *sam* in Cantonese (in other Cantonese dialects, it is pronounced *sin*, same as for the word 線, meaning "Line" or "Thread"). This may be where much of the confusion between Centerline and Centerline Plane has stemmed from as 中心 literally means "center to the heart" or "center of the heart." It also means the "core" or "center core." It further has the meaning of "focus" and "concentration." So, for Chinese Wing Chun practitioners, 中心 actually refers to a lot more than just a vertical line drawn superficially on the center front of a human figure, which is what most Western practitioners of Wing Chun think of. When you look at the 中 symbol face on, you can see how the rectangular body is divided in half, which can symbolize how our bodies are divided into two sagittal sides. Being aware of (and utilizing) these two sides independently and interdependently is a very important factor in one's Wing Chun training.

The character has a further meaning as well, representing the state of middle way or neutrality. Buddhism teaches one to take the middle path and not veer towards extremes. In Wing Chun, one must remain neutral mentally, physically and emotionally. Doing so will allow the practitioner to shift to either side of the scale when necessary, and yet still retain the ability to return to the middle. Chinese characters don't have circular or "S" shaped symbols, therefore the 中 character can be said to represent a curved line in the middle of a circle, such as the Yin-Yang symbol, indicating the need for harmony between two independent yet interdependent entities. As we've seen, the concept of Wing Chun is very much intertwined with the philosophy of Yin-Yang.

Looking at 中 from a bird's-eye view one can see how the vertical line represents the Centerline Plane passing through the center of a body. In Wing Chun it is very important to understand not only what the Centerline means, but also to recognize that the Centerline Plane (中線) joins your Centerline to that of your opponent. The Chinese characters 中心, meaning "center," "central," "centerline," "center core," "mindfulness," "focus," "focusing centrally," "concentration," "middle," or "neutral," takes on a different meaning when the heart symbol is replaced by another character. When it is replaced by 線, meaning "line," "path" or "plane," it could mean "center (vertical) line," "center (horizontal) line," "centerline," "centerline plane," "center plane" or "center path." In Wing Chun, the vertical line that runs from the apex of your head (前頂, *Qianding*, meaning Front Crown of Head) through the center core of your upper torso to the middle of your perineum (會陰, Huiyin, meaning the Yin Convergence Point) is called *cheong sam sin* (中心線), or just *cheong sam*; roughly translated into English as the "Centerline" or "Center Core." Whereas the path that runs from one Centerline to another is called *cheong sin* (中線), or roughly translated to English as the "Centerline Plane."

It is vital for Wing Chun practitioners to understand that the Centerline runs inside the body—not outside of it. Because many practitioners think of the Centerline as something external, they additionally mark centerlines for the back and sides of the body. This is unnecessary when you come to view the Centerline as being situated in the center core of the body. Knowing this, you can target your opponent's Centerline from any angle and, by the same token, you can protect your own Centerline from any angle when facing your opponent. Additionally, when you focus on the center core of your opponent, you will be able to strike through the surface of his body to hit it, whereas if you look at the Centerline as being merely an external mark on the surface of your opponent's body, your mind will tend to target it superficially.

One of the primary objectives of training in Wing Chun is to make the practitioner fully aware of both his own Centerline and that of his opponent's, in addition to the Centerline path that connects his Centerline to that of his opponent's. With this awareness, the practitioner can focus on attacking his opponent's Centerline along the Centerline path, while protecting his own Centerline along the Centerline path. This type of focus and awareness must not slip away for a moment.

In Wing Chun, there are other vocabularies stemming from 中心 (*cheong sam*) that are associated with the training. For example, when the character for "center" (中) is replaced by the character for "inner feelings" (衷), the new combination (衷心—*cung sam*) translates as "wholehearted" or "wholeheartedly." When the character for "center" (中) is replaced by the character meaning "loyal," "devoted" or "honest" (忠), the new combination (忠心–*zung sam*) now translates as "devotion" or "dedication."

There is a saying in Wing Chun that, "A punch starts from the heart," which many practitioners take literally by placing their fist in front of their heart as a starting point for their punch. With the understanding of what 心, 中心, 衷心, and 忠心 means, we can now better interpret this as "punch with focus," "punch with concentrated force," "punch wholeheartedly," "punch from the center," "punch to the center," "punch from the core," or "punch to the core." In Mandarin, all three combinations (中心, 衷心 and 忠心) are pronounced the same; *troong shin* (*zhong xin* in the Pinyin Romanization). So, when a Chinese teacher tells his student to "practice with *troong shin*," it can mean to "practice with focus," or "practice with devotion," or "practice wholeheartedly," or all three together.

When you understand the Chinese language, the Centerline principle takes on a whole different and much deeper meaning than what is typically presented in most books and articles on this Wing Chun principle. In order to master Wing Chun a student must be very centered, focused, devoted, dedicated, and true to himself. This is the main principle of Wing Chun from which all other principles and attributes arise. Without these core characteristics, a practitioner would never be able to attain any of the goals he set out to reach.

THE IMPORTANCE OF HAVING GOALS

A Wing Chun practitioner should have a goal. This goal could be anything from becoming a master of the art, to merely reaching a certain level of proficiency in the art, to unlocking the secrets to better understanding the art, to teaching the art, to maintaining one's health, to building one's character, to overcoming mental challenges, to overcoming physical challenges—to achieving all of these things. In order to accomplish these objectives the practitioner must raise his consciousness to a higher level. He must learn what his limitations and capabilities are. He must know that he or she has the potential to improve dramatically and even to be the best in whatever endeavor he or she chooses to take on. The Wing Chun practitioner must learn to prioritize the communication between mind and body; to isolate (or unite) parts of the mind and body as needed. The Wing Chun practitioner must realize that each part of the body has its own independent role and yet must still be able to coordinate with other parts of the body when necessary. When the practitioner encounters an opponent or an opposing force, he will need to overcome it with the mental and physical skills that he has acquired in his training. The mental skills will involve the ability to focus relentlessly on the little details as well as the big issues, and to know how to prioritize these effectively. This will involve a new way of thinking that is different from the norm. By the same token, it will involve freeing the mind from clutter and confusion, thus enabling it to scan the problem clearly and quickly piece together the various bits of information required to resolve the situation. In order to do this, however, there must exist a strong connection between the mind and body; a very efficient and effective two-way communication must be present. There must not be any lag time between the brain receiving a message and the body responding with physical action. The physical action will involve the coordination of many body parts or the isolation of one single part for one single action, or the combination of two or more parts for a single action; or the combination of two or more parts for a dual or triple action; or the prioritization of different parts of the body to act sequentially for a single action, or the prioritization of different parts of the body to act sequentially for a dual or triple action. Furthermore, it will involve the enhancement of acute tactile senses to read the opponent's actions accurately, and to develop the ability to instantly transmit messages to the mind for immediate response.

The Wing Chun training program is multi-faceted. The forms, exercises, and drills manifest the goals and strategies of the system. When understood and practiced properly, the program will help each practitioner reach his or her own goals and objectives. It will also help the practitioner develop the proper emotion and spirit that are required for him to attain them. These are vital components required (in addition to mental and physical strength) in order for one to successfully overcome obstacles, resolve conflicts and to win battles.

Now all of this will sound like so much jargon to those people who don't comprehend the concept of reading an opponent's force and movements through the sense of touch, and by those who assert themselves against their opponents too aggressively and speedily. Such people may well be aware of their own actions, but they will have no clue about the significance of their opponent's actions. This is where the concept of Chisau, "sticking hands," comes into play, which I refer to as "the science of espionage."

NINE

CHISAU: THE SCIENCE OF ESPIONAGE

WING CHUN'S CHISAU EXERCISE is unique to the art. It is vastly different from the energy/tactile development exercises that one may find in other Chinese martial arts such as Tai Chi and Bagua. In these arts there is an exercise called "Push-Hands," that requires their practitioners to touch arms in order to detect their opponent's strengths, weaknesses and the direction of his movements—but "Push-Hands" is very different from Chisau.

HUMAN SENSORY SYSTEMS

Of the five senses, two are particularly acute—the senses of sight and touch, while the remaining senses are not as keenly developed as those of animals, birds, reptiles, and insects. However, all of our senses are working at all times, continuously delivering messages to our conscious or subconscious mind. Our senses transmit information to our brain about everything in our environment and they are particularly helpful to us in detecting threats to our wellbeing, and alerting us to potential danger and its proximity. However, in a panic situation, many people seem to disconnect from their sensory feedback mechanisms, resulting in a loss of control of even their sense of sight and touch; things can begin to look blurry and feel numb.

The Wing Chun concept, along with its training program, trains people to bring their visual and tactile senses to an absolute peak of development and also to keep their brains in constant contact with all of their senses in order to heighten total awareness during a combative situation. Wing Chun views our senses as transmissions from our central and peripheral nervous systems. We do not consider our eyes as something separate from our skin or the rest of our bodies. All of our senses work together to report on the goings on both within our own bodies and within our immediate environment. And with proper training, one's mind will be sharpened to receive crystal clear visual and tactile information even under the most intense situations.

Musashi, in his *Book of Five Rings*, describes what type of gaze you must have when facing and fighting an opponent:

"You should gaze largely and widely. This is a gaze of perception and sight. The perception should be strong, and sight should be weak."

Musashi's book relates how one should focus one's vision widely and narrowly, and see small things big and big things small, and to have peripheral vision without shifting one's eyes. He instructs his student to practice this gaze in daily life.

When performing Chisau many Wing Chun practitioners will tend to look away from their partner in the belief that by taking the sense of sight out of the equation they will have to rely more on their sense of touch, and that practicing this way will really heighten or improve their tactile sense, which they wish to be as acute as possible in the event they should get into a real fight. While the desire to improve one's tactile sensitivity is a good thing, looking away from your partner during training is never a good idea; it will condition you to do so in a real encounter, which would be a foolhardy thing to do in a life-or-death situation. In such a situation every sense can play an important role in your survival and can assist you in getting out of a potentially life-threatening situation. To use anything less than all of your senses in such an encounter would be to needlessly handicap yourself and diminish your chances for survival.

With this in mind it is imperative that one trains all of one's senses in order to cultivate *maximum* acuity. Training the visual sense in particular should be a top priority, as the eyes must be trained to perceive more than just mere images. You must be able to gaze into the eyes of your opponent, the focal point of your strike, and through to your opponent's Centerline core without shifting your eyes.

In my Qigong training, I exercise my internal organs by seeing them in my mind and then casting them far away and bouncing them back. If a person well-trained in Wing Chun intends to strike at his opponent's heart, he will gaze into his opponent's chest, see his heart and strike it. Skilled acupuncturists do this as well; they need to "see" where their needle is penetrating in order to connect with the appropriate meridian and not hit a vital organ. This type of seeing is no different than the one employed by golfers who can "see the hole" and the most efficient route to it from a distance away, and then direct the ball to it by that route. To cultivate this ability in Wing Chun, it is very important to understand how and where to direct your visual attention when performing the various forms or when engaged in Chisau.

The primary objective of the Chisau exercise is to bring your sense of touch up to its highest level of sensitivity so that you will have additional help in reading your opponent's intentions when fighting him. Sun Tzu wrote:

> If you know the enemy and know yourself, you need not fear the result of a hundred battles. If you know yourself but not the enemy, for every victory gained, you will also suffer a defeat. If you know neither your enemy nor yourself, you will succumb in every battle.

This is precisely the strategy underlying Chisau training; i.e., to know your opponent and to know yourself through the tactile energy feedback you receive through your sense of touch.

The sense of vision obviously plays a huge role in a combative situation, allowing combatants to detect one another's movements in defense and attack. However, since most people use their sense of sight in a fight, then neither one has a sensory advantage over the other. And if one of the combatants has a natural advantage in physical size over another combatant, a one-to-one match up of skills will not help the smaller person to overcome the larger one. Developing one's tactile sense to a higher degree than one's opponent, however, will give one a decided (and additional) advantage. Not only will this sense act as a supplement to your visual sense, but it will become your main data receiver should your vision become obstructed, blurred or directed elsewhere. Your arms and hands can be likened to the antennae of insects probing for information or as spies that you have placed in enemy territory to extract information and send it back to headquarters.

In the Wing Chun training program Chisau is practiced for the following reasons:

1. To make one's arms more sensitive to incoming and outgoing energy.
2. To train one to understand the boundaries of the body.

3. To align incoming and outgoing forces to both heels or to the heel of the rear leg (where the majority of the body's weight should be carried).
4. To assigning certain responsibilities to each arm and each section of the arm.
5. And most importantly, to develop the mind to reach a higher level of consciousness.

When the above is achieved, it becomes easy to control and trap an opponent's arms and then to attack him at will. Unfortunately, I have seldom witnessed this skill fully cultivated in most Wing Chun schools. Instead they engage in an activity of rolling their arms aggressively, and then suddenly breaking away to throw multiple uncontrolled strikes.

In the Chisau trapping exercise, the practitioner learns that there are only four possible ways that one's arms can engage with both of the opponent's arms:

1. When both of one's arms are within both of the opponent's arms.
2. When both of one's arms are outside both of the opponent's arms.
3. When one's right arm is inside, and one's left is outside of the opponent's opposite arms.
4. When one's left arm is inside, and one's right arm is outside of the opponent's opposite arms.

Wing Chun then teaches several ways to deal or trap-attack the opponent from these four positions, giving one the advantage of being aware of these positions and then developing reactions from them. This is not to say that you should go searching for your opponent's arms in order to get into these positions, but it is important that you be aware of them when you find your arms to be in any of these positions, and to react accordingly.

Certainly, there will be situations when one's arms will not be in contact with the opponent's arms, or that just one arm is in contact with one of the opponent's arms. These are common occurrences when one's concept of fighting is to keep a "safe" distance, and to move in for an attack and retreat immediately back to the safe distance, and to use just one arm at a time to strike or block, with no concern to read the opponent's actions through the tactile sense, as is done with boxing or many other martial arts. Wing Chun concept of fighting is to make contact with the opponent immediately with both arms (and one leg), and to attack and defend using both arms (and leg) simultaneously. The four possible entanglements listed above occur when both arms are used to engage the opponent's both arms;

however, if no contact is made, the visual sense takes priority; if one contact is made, then that will be used to read the opponent's force and action.

Wing Chun is not the only martial art that has the concept of reading the opponent's actions through tactile sense. Tai Chi, Bagua, Jujitsu, Judo, Aikido, and wrestling do the same. These arts are heavily dependent on arm or body contact. Wing Chun does not only use the arm to sense the opponent's force and actions, but uses all parts of the body to do it. The Chisau exercise not only sensitizes the arms, but the whole body. The arms are used just as a means to develop higher consciousness. It is the mind that is getting trained, not the arms. During the Chisau exercise, the practitioner must use the contact point to feel the opponent's whole body, if not at least the one sagittal side of the opponent's body where the contact is made. By the same token, the practitioner must feel his own whole body, if not at least the one sagittal side of his body where the contact is made. The feeling should be like an electric current that runs through the whole body when a contact is made, and to make it go wherever the practitioner wants it to go—particularly to the ground, through the heels. This is how you'd become one with your opponent or training partner. You'd then dance with him just like Ginger Rogers did with Fred Astaire. Note that I put Ginger's name ahead of Fred's because she's the one who was required to read his momentous and fast movements, and then respond in real-time (or milliseconds behind) without noticeable lag.

There are several levels of Chisau progression. With patience, slow practice, and trusting both the art and the teacher, a practitioner will master each level in progression. However, most practitioners, including many well-known ones, never even reach the first level of proficiency even after years of practice. Once the Wing Chun practitioner has mastered a certain level of proficiency with his hands, he or she will (or should) be taught *Chigerk*— the counterpart of Chisau— using just one's legs.

In Chisau the focus should be on utilizing both arms. Singular actions, although common and necessary, are not really emphasized in Wing Chun. The belief is that anyone can throw a punch with one arm that is followed by another, or block an incoming attack and then counter with a strike. You needn't teach anyone to do that. Most people have the common sense and simple survival instinct to respond in such a manner. However, if you programmed two robots to fight in this way they would never hit each other; Robot A would throw a kick while Robot B would block the kick and then throw a punch, which Robot A would block—and on and on it would go. Wing Chun is an art that was developed for human beings—not robots.

Whether you are engaged in a war, or playing chess or football, a good strategy with multiple options will always better your chances of securing a victory. In Wing Chun, one of the strategies we use is to trap and immobilize the opponent before making our final move. Such an action ensures minimum risk and maximizes our chance of success. As a result, the Wing Chun fighting concept encourages trapping movements. This can only be executed successfully, however, when one can clearly read the intentions, strengths, weaknesses and actions of the opponent, which, in the case of Wing Chun practitioners, comes from the diligent practice of both Chisau and Chigerk.

TEN

Structure: The Science of Architecture

I HAVE MENTIONED EARLIER THE importance of "structure" in Wing Chun. Now let us examine this concept in greater detail. The human body is a complex mechanism. Bio-scientists don't have all the answers yet, but they've already come light years in understanding many different aspects of the human body such as its anatomy, energy and muscular systems and its architecture.

Recently, there has been a focus on the architecture of the body and its kinesiology; that is, the science of how the body is designed and structured, and how it moves. One of the newest discoveries is that the human body is wired tensionally in a dynamic self-supportive manner that allows for omi-directional movement, and that it can adjust to fortify its structure in such a way so as to utilize less energy and yet enhance mobility. The word used to describe this theorem is called *biotensegrity*, which was coined by Stephen Levin MD in 1980.

BIOTENSEGRITY

The term *biotensegrity* is a word that you will not find in a standard dictionary. It is made up of the prefix "bio," as in biology or the science of life; "tense," as in tension; and "grity," as in integrity. The term *tensegrity* was minted by Richard Buckminster Fuller (1895-1983), an American engineer, designer, and architect. In fact, he designed the Geodesic Dome for the US pavilion at Expo '67 in Montreal, Canada. Currently, you will find geodesic domes in Ontario Place in Toronto, and the Science Center in Vancouver. These domes have no internal supports, and are made up of interlocking triangular shaped structures. The tetrahedrons (four-sided pyramids of equilateral angles) form a three-way hemispherical grid that distributes support stress evenly to the entire structure, therefore rendering a very high strength-to-weight ratio.

Only in recent history have bioscientists recognized tension forces in the human structure. The general consensus had been based on the axial-loaded compression support system, that is, bones in the spinal column are stacked one on top of each other, and are held together by muscles and gravity. The problem with such a structure is that it can be pulled apart by the forces that hold them together if slightly tilted. The stacked vertebrate model is only useful when it is perfectly balanced, upright and immobile. In the horizontal position of a four-legged animal such as an elephant or large Bengal tiger, the spine wouldn't be able to withstand the muscular weight and the force of gravity. Even the weight of the head when tilted on top of the spine would be too much to bear for a person. It would be impossible for a person to bend, reach out, or lift objects. Muscle alone couldn't lift moderate weights, especially when the load extends away from the body. Biologic structures, however, are mobile, flexibly hinged, low-energy consuming, omnidirectional in movement, and can function free of gravity. While architectural columns bear loads only from above, the spine can accept loads from any direction. The spine can bend forward, backward, sideways; twist and bend simultaneously; and perform gymnastics, dances, or martial arts in any environment.

The newest theory of the human structure is based on a class of trusses called "tensegrity." The tensegrity-structured spinal column suspends in a network of tensed muscles, tendons, ligaments, and tissues, much like how the hub of a bicycle's wired wheel suspends in a network of tensed spokes. Such structure is applicable to bipeds or quadrupeds, in supine, prone, or upside down position, in any environment. The human shoulder girdle is made up of a pair of scapulae, and a pair of clavicles. The scapula, known in layman's terms as the shoulder blade, does not press against the thorax or the spine. The clavicle (collar bone) connects one end to the sternum, and the other end to the scapula. The humerus (upper arm) fits into the socket of the scapula. Without direct support from the spinal column, how do the arms, shoulder and collarbone support loads twice the amount of our own weight?

There is no doubt that the tensegrity system plays a very significant role in the support of the shoulder girdle. Also, there is no doubt that the pelvis is involved in all bodily movement. Like the shoulder socket, at the end of the hipbone is a cavity called the acetabulum, and this is where the femur (thighbone) fits. The weight of the trunk transfers from the spine, through the sacrum, through the hipbone to the thighbone, and from there onto the lower leg and foot. Conversely, all forces acting on the lower limbs are transmitted to the trunk by the same route.

Understanding how the biotensegrity structure works will help us to better understand how our ligaments, tendons and muscles work when applying our Wing Chun movements. Our ligaments, tendons and the inner muscles are always under tension. There is, of course, a tension range—from minimum to maximum. The minimum is the resting length and the maximum is the farthest length they will stretch before they tear. However, the soft tissues are very strong and can withstand a tremendous amount of tension. This formula is readily observed operating in the movements of Wing Chun and in other martial arts. In Wing Chun, one often will receive the incoming force from an opponent's strike via a pelvic rotation before striking out with one's own force via a counter rotation of the pelvis. This type of force—going from zero pelvic position to a -45 degree rotational position before rotating to a +45 degree position—is much stronger than simply going from a 0 degree to a +45 degree position. Obviously, you've rotated 90 degrees in the former example versus only 45 degrees in the latter. Not only that, but the principle of tensegrity goes to work in doubling that force. In other words, when the tension elements are twisted (i.e., tension is increased), the resulting action is a counter twist to return to the resting length.

Since the scapula is not directly pressed against the spine, load transfer does not occur directly from the scapula to the spine. Rather, the loads or forces are transferred via a network of tensed intertwined ligaments and inner and smaller muscles. Therefore, a push or a punch is not dependent (or entirely dependent) on the force of gravity, but mainly on the tensegrity system. A pull is not dependent on a lever system alone, but on tensegrity as well. If a punch were totally dependent on gravitational force alone, our bones and structure would not be able to withstand the impact from the reaction force. However, in a tensegrity system, the network of ligaments and soft tissues are able to absorb and distribute the impact throughout the network in a balanced manner.

To "throw" a fast punch, the ligaments and small muscles must be pliable, flexible, and resilient. Their power comes from the amount of velocity generated by the effort (muscles involved in the movement), and the counter reaction of the receiving mass against the leverage. In other words, the receiving mass in this instance is your opponent, a set of boards or bricks, and the leverage comes from the ground you push against, your back, or your arm alone (whatever you use for leverage). The power you generate from a punch is caused by the interrelationship of your tensegrity elements (the ligaments and small tissues), much like using a rubber band to strike an object; that is, from resting length to fully stretched length to rebounding past the resting length, to final resting length.

Tensegrity works on the principle of a network of flexible elements. In the human body, the ligaments, tendons, small muscles, and tissues make up the tensegrity network. The bigger superficial muscles, such as the calves, biceps, pectoralis major and latissimus doris, although also a part of the tensegrity network, function more towards compression work, much like the tire on a bicycle wheel (with the bones serving as a rim). A rigid cartwheel consisting of 3 or 4 rigid spokes does not constitute a tensegrity system. This is a very important factor to understand for Wing Chun and other martial arts.

For the human body, the ligaments, tendons and small muscular tissues mainly make up the tensegrity network. Ligaments are bands of slightly elastic tissues that hold ends of bones at the joints together. They are more elastic than tendons, but less elastic than muscles. Tendons are located at the ends of muscles and serve to anchor muscles to the bones. Tendon cells regenerate very slowly and are very inelastic; muscles, by contrast, are very elastic; their cells regenerate easily. Muscle tissue is made up of fibers, which hold the muscles together.

When one injures one's ligaments or tendons, biomechanical doctors prescribe strength training for the patient in order to strengthen the surrounding, supporting musculature, because the larger and stronger muscles serve to dissipate stress from the ligaments and tendons. In other words, the muscles take up the job of the ligaments and tendons. While this is a good prescription for preventing and rehabilitating an injury, it is not quite as beneficial for tensegrity dependent actions. Because muscles regenerate easily and quickly, muscle buildup is visibly evident. In bodybuilding, for instance, one's muscles are torn down to some degree and then repaired and made a little bigger and stronger. Through special diet, this process of regeneration is enhanced, resulting in the muscles being built up larger. However, if muscles are built up too large a certain degree of elasticity will be lost—not all of it, of course, but some degree of plasticity will be compromised for sure. What happens when the ligaments and tendons almost lose their jobs?

The spokes of a bicycle or motorcycle wheel in a tensegrity system spread the load applied on the hub to the whole rim. The air-filled tire works on the same principle. Instead of spokes, air acts as the tensegrity element to push against the inside of the tire evenly at every point. The compression/load where the tire meets the ground is spread evenly throughout the whole tire. On the other hand, the ancient wagon cartwheel, designed as a circular lever system, depended totally on the size and strength of the rim and the strength of the solid spoke that was directly underneath the wheel's axle at a given time for its support. In other words, the spokes were designed only to hold the frame of the wheel and to support the wagon when a spoke was directly underneath the axle. When one spoke bore the weight of the wagon, the other spokes were free from compression. So, the larger and heavier a wagon was, the larger and thicker a cartwheel was required. They were not very strong, however, even when they had 12 spokes, since they were rigid and were based on a lever system. You no doubt have seen enough Cowboy movies over the years to know that these cartwheels almost always broke when they were made to move faster over uneven ground.

Large and hard muscles work very much like the cartwheel; they take over the workload and minimize the work of the tensegrity network. Proper weight training is good for general health and strength building, but a buildup of too much muscle will cause a loss of elasticity, thus lessening the functionality of the ligaments, tendons and smaller muscles. The increase in muscle mass would also require more energy to engage these muscles. Remember, force is directly related to mass, energy, and motion. In Physics, force is only considered when an action or influence accelerates an object. If you are standing still and push against a wall, and there is no move-ment, then there is zero net force, or that the force that you've generated and counter generated are in an equilibrium state; however, if you run into a wall and are bounced back from it, then the equal and opposite force that both you and the wall generated accounts for the force. So, when you push an object, and use ten units of energy, you will require twenty units of energy to move an object twice the mass. If you use ten units of energy to push the larger mass, the acceleration will be reduced by 50 percent.

As indicated earlier, ligament and tendon cells regenerate very slowly, unlike muscles. When you tear a muscle, your system quickly repairs and rebuilds it. This is possible because blood runs through muscles to supply oxygen and nutrients. On the other hand, blood does not run through lig-aments and tendons at the same rate as it does muscles. Thus, should you damage a ligament or tendon, it takes a long time to heal—if it heals at all.

In all areas of life there is always a tradeoff and it's in the nature of things that if you concentrate on only one factor, the scale will tip in that direction. There is a principle in exercise physiology known as the S.A.I.D. Principle, which stands for Specific Adaptation to Imposed Demands. The principle states, essentially, that your body will adapt specifically to what you are doing in the way you are doing it. Change what you are doing or the way you are doing it, and another adaptation must be made. For example, if bodybuilding is your passion, then (genetics permitting) the time and effort you expend in building muscle mass will see your body use 100 percent of its adaptive energy for improving your muscle building efforts. If your passion is martial arts, then the time and effort you expend in practicing the martial arts will see your body use 100 percent of its adaptive energy for improving your martial arts skills. However, if you do attempt to do both and give both an equal amount of time and effort, you won't get 100 percent adaptive benefit in both. It's not like there exists 100 units of adaptation energy for martial arts and another 100 units of adaptation energy for bodybuilding (or piano playing, or football, etc.); there exists 100 units of adaptation energy—period. So if you devote yourself to bodybuilding and martial arts equally, then your adaptation energy will be 50–50 in both. If you split up your time and energy investment 70–30, then you'll get 70–30 results; and if you split it 30–70, you will get 30–70. Arnold Schwarzenegger concentrated solely on bodybuilding to win his seven Mr. Olympia titles. Bruce Lee concentrated on martial arts to become the King of martial arts. Because of the amount of muscle he built, Schwarzenegger would never be able to punch as fast as Lee or hit as hard as Lee did. Conversely, Lee would not have been able to push as much weight or build as much muscle mass as Schwarzenegger. Although speed is not everything in martial arts, it is definitely a prerequisite; however, it is not required in bodybuilding.

When we're not in motion, our bodies' tensegrity elements are at their resting length. This position can be considered a neutral position. Our muscles are in cross-pattern for the purpose of tensegrity efficiency. When our arms hang down to our sides, they're in a neutral tensegrity position, but when you rotate your arm clockwise or anti-clockwise this movement stretches the tensegrity elements. You will agree with me that if we walked around with our arms fully twisted all day our arms would be very tired by the end of the day. The tensegrity system will always want the elements to return to resting length and any position other than the neutral position will result in a taxing of the tensegrity elements.

I believe the developers of Wing Chun recognized this, and opted for a vertical-positioned fist (rather than the horizontal-position fist as in most other arts) because of this fact. A twisted or horizontal (pronated) hand would only cause resistance and stress to the arm and diminish the potency of the punch. Relaxed muscles, whereby there is minimal tension placed on the ligaments and tendons, always produces the most effective punch in terms of speed and power.

I'm convinced more than ever that the developers of Wing Chun were scientific geniuses—physicists, kinesiologists and martial artists of the highest caliber. Although they didn't coin the word biotensegrity, they knew exactly how the human body worked and they then set about designing a martial art system that reflected the design and systems of the human body; that is, a system that had simplicity and complexity intertwined to deliver maximum diversity from minimum inventory.

THE SACRUM—THE HUB OF POWER

The sacroiliac joint (the joint between the sacrum and the ilium, or upper portion of the hipbone) connects the pelvis to the spine.

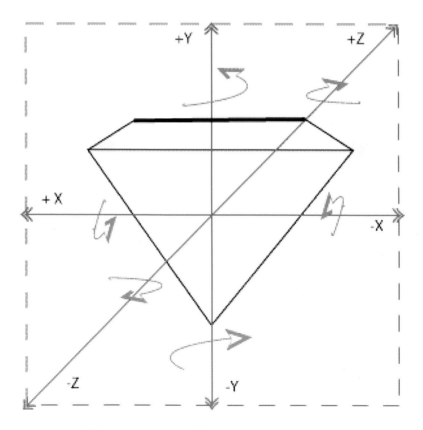

The sacrum rotates around three axis points—X, Y, and Z.

[95]

The sacrum does not behave as a keystone, but quite the opposite. The sacrum and the spine above it slings in the pelvis rather than compresses into the pelvis.

The sacrum has six degrees (or 12 degrees, consisting of six positive and six negative degrees) of free movement in a 3-D Cartesian coordinate system; i.e., rotating around three axis points—X, Y and Z. (See Illustration 10-1). Fuller proved that for any tensegrity structure, twelve restraints are required to fix a point in space. It takes just twelve tension spokes to rigidly fix the hub of a bicycle wheel in space; the extra spokes are placed only for fail-safe backup. The hub is fixed in its tension network and the compression loads are distributed around the rim. In the human biotensegrity structure, the pelvis ring is the rim, and the sacrum is the hub. The ligaments and muscles that attach the sacrum to the pelvis ring are the tension elements. The loads are transferred through the tension network, thus allowing for omnidirectional stability that is independent of gravity. Therefore, even when a person shifts his weight or stands on one leg, the sacrum remains fixed just as the bicycle's hub of the wheel does when it is on just one wheel.

When the sacrum moves in tandem with other bones of the pelvis, as in rotating or shifting movements, the ligaments remain at the same length in a tension-coupled pattern. The crossed ligament pattern exists in the spine, at the disc, the hip, the back, sacroiliac joints, iliolumbar, and other muscles and soft tissues of the pelvis-spine-hip network. Our spinal ligaments are never relaxed; they are always tense, at least in resting length. The ligaments act as rubber-bands; they stretch, but return to their resting length. The muscles attached to the spine are also in a state of tension.

TRIANGULATION

Triangulated structures are inherently stable. Structures that are not triangulated, such as a square, have joints that must be rigidly fixed to keep from collapsing. These joints generate torque and bending effects and have high-energy requirements. A square frame structure is only stable when forces (compression) pass through the joints perpendicular to the joints.

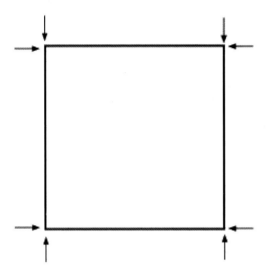

A square frame is only stable when forces pass through the joints perpendicularly.

If the frame is made of non-rigid material, such as a rope, then bending will occur when forces are applied to the joints, as torque is being created at the joints.

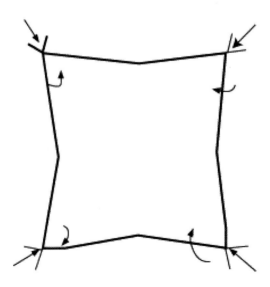

When forces are applied to the joints of a square frame that is non-rigid, it will bend.

When force is applied from another angle, the structure will shear.

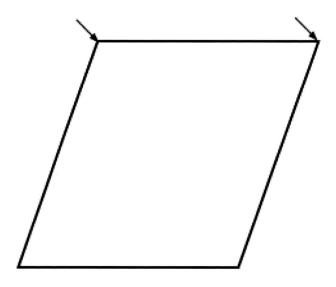

A square frame will shear when force is applied from an angle.

Triangles are stable with flexible joints and have no torque or bending effects at the joints. There are only tension and compression members in a triangle; therefore triangles are low energy consumers. However, a triangular frame of non-rigid material will remain stable as the elements are either in tension or compression, and free of torque at the joints.

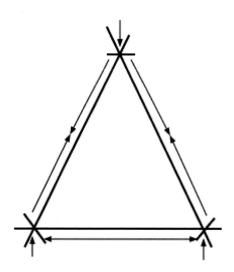

A non-rigid triangular frame is stable because the elements are free of torque at the joints.

The laws of evolution and the laws of nature are intimately related to the laws of triangulation and close-packing configuration for space and energy efficiency. The beehive is hexagonally configured for close packing; graphite is also hexagonally packed with carbon atoms; diamonds, one of the hardest materials on earth, are packed with carbon atoms in a tetrahedral configuration; methane and water molecules are also configured as tetrahedrons. Closely packed icosahedrons are fully triangulated and make the most spherical and symmetrical polyhedron.

Whether we are products of creation or evolution, we had to be cleverly and efficiently designed or evolved from selections of the best systems. It is believed that we are linked in a hierarchical construction that starts at the smallest sub-cellular component and builds itself like a beehive. Our structure is one integrated tensegrity truss that evolves from infinitely smaller trusses that could be structurally independent and interdependent at the same time. Doesn't this remind you of the Yin-Yang philosophy?

The truss design that fits these requirements is the icosahedron, i.e., a geometric figure that has twenty sides or planes. The outer shell is under tension and the vertices are held apart by internal compression struts that suspend in a tension network. The compression elements do not press on one another, but rather are fixed in position by the tension network. The tensegrity icosahedron is a fully triangulated three-dimensional truss. It is an omnidirectional, gravity independent, flexible hinged structure whose mechanical behavior is non-linear. It is stable even with frictionless hinges, and can be altered in shape or stiffness merely by shortening and lengthening one or several tension elements.

When a tensegrity icosahedron is viewed as a model for the skeletal system, the bones are seen as the compressive elements, and the soft tissues as the tension elements, with the result that the structure will be stable in any position, even with multiple joints. When movement is created, or one tissue is shortened, a rippling effect runs through the structure, creating a new stable shape that is low-energy consuming, highly mobile, and omnidirectional. The sacroiliac joint and the scapulothoracic joint are involved in our lower and upper movements. These joints are at play mostly in the art of Wing Chun but also in several other internal-oriented martial arts. Understanding how they are structured and work will make one understand their maximum potential and weakest link. It is just as the Principle of Whole System states, that knowing or discovering a part and its behavior makes it possible for the discovery of the presence of other parts and behavior. To know Wing Chun as a whole system, one needs to know each part and its behavior. Knowing human structure and its behavior is an essential part of knowing Wing Chun.

[99]

The pelvic complex is a self-organizing structure that is part of a larger, fractal, closely packed tensegrity structure that integrates with other parts into the whole. The Wing Chun founders followed this principle in designing the Wing Chun fighting system and training method—amalgamating simplicity and complexity to deliver minimum inventory with maximum diversity. Each design or movement was closely packed, integrating with other parts into a greater whole.

Many refer to Wing Chun as a linear fighting system, but in actuality it takes on any geometric shape and path to accomplish the combative objective in the most economical, efficient and productive way. However, it uses the triangular shape more than the others because of the triangle's ability to fit into any other geometric shape. Although Wing Chun movements take linear paths, they are not done singularly. What sets Wing Chun apart from other fighting systems is the simultaneous usage of two or three limbs for a defense-offense action. A skilled Wing Chun practitioner would never execute a single block, a single arm strike, or a single kick. Those Wing Chun sifus pictured in the magazines throwing a sidekick above waist height are misrepresenting Wing Chun. What you are seeing there is syncretic Wing Chun.

Although the movements in the Wing Chun forms are performed singularly (particularly in the Siu Nim Tau form), they were originally designed to help the practitioner understand and practice each movement perfectly. However, when it comes to Chisau, sparring, or fighting, they are to be used in conjunction.

I have earlier pointed out how the Centerline concept is one of Wing Chun's primary principles and how it trains the practitioner to focus his attacks toward his opponent's Centerline. Since our arms extend from our shoulder joints, we naturally form a triangle when we use both of our arms simultaneously to attack an opponent's Centerline. The triangle takes on different shapes, depending on the angle of our body relative to that of the opponent. The formation of the triangle by the arms can act as deflectors against attacks directed to our Centerline by the opponent. Also, attacking the opponent's Centerline along our Centerline Plane will deliver a much more powerful hit than attacking anywhere else because the returned force can be absorbed by the spine (the main support structure for the upper torso) and transferred to the ground through the legs, and returned back to the opponent again. For our lower trunk, the legs and feet in the Yijikim Yeungma position create the triangular shapes. When stepping forward, the foot moves toward the opponent's Centerline, and the triangular component is maintained to ensure stability and security. Similarly, when you use your foot to kick, it moves toward the opponent's Centerline; you bend your knee to maintain the triangular component for stability and security.

YIJIKIM YEUNGMA

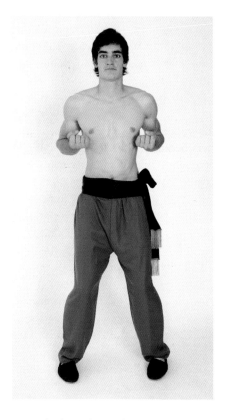
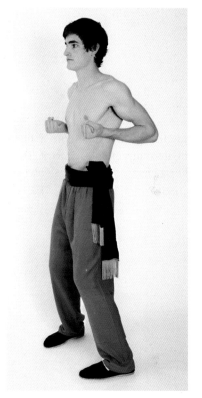

Wing Chun's Fundamental Horse—Yijikim
Yeungma (front view)

Yijikim Yeungma (diagonal view)

The Yijikim Yeungma is a structurally strong and balanced posture. A person's legs in this posture are directly underneath and within the parameters of the upper torso, and so are able to support it with little effort (energy from muscular use) and stress (on the joints)—much like a typical relaxed posture when one is standing in line waiting for a bus. When you are in a relaxed stance; i.e., your feet are shoulder-width apart, you could probably stack ten people on your shoulders, one atop of each other, as long as they line up with the Line of Gravity (LoG). The design of your tensegrity structure will hold them without you having to use any additional muscular force. The ten guys could even cantilever from the LoG sideways as long as the two sides pull on each other to form a tensegrity structure—as can be witnessed in displays of acrobats. The wide and low riding stances in Karate, Taekwondo, and some Kung Fu arts are overrated for strength and balance; because when one's thighs cantilever past the upper torso and one's knees are bent at an angle near 90 degrees, there is a lot of stress put on one's pelvic joints and knees. A person in this posture would have trouble stacking two guys on his shoulders because all his leg muscles will be working very hard simply to hold this position even without the extra load. The original idea behind assuming a wide stance was to create a wide base to enhance one's stability and balance. However, it is utterly immobile, very taxing on the muscles, and not nearly as strong a stance as was originally believed.

In Wing Chun, the 6.5-Pole form uses a low riding stance, but only to exercise and strengthen the legs rather than as a fighting stance. I suppose it could possibly be used in fighting—I'm stretching a bit here—perhaps as a finishing position when delivering a side punch to an opponent's ribs or solar plexus and a lunge is required to cover the distance. However, I believe that most of the low stances in the other martial arts were also originally developed for leg exercise but that this somehow got lost in translation and eventually these postures were made into fighting stances. If anyone believes that a low stance is functional for fighting, just try sparring in it. Of all the sparring and competitions I've seen, I've never seen anyone stand that low when fighting—even by the practitioners of arts that train with such low stances.

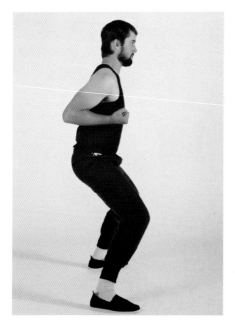

The classic Horse-Riding stance

The Yijikim Yeungma is very much a natural stance with a slight deviation. The thighs are parallel to each other and aligned with each sagittal side of the upper torso like a natural stance, however, the lower legs angle out to form a brace from the ground to the knees. The feet are pigeon-toed to create a triangular shape, with a wider base at the back to withstand frontal forces. The beauty of this stance is that when you need to lower yourself to absorb a frontal force or lower your center of gravity, the thighs squeeze inward rather than cantilever out of the upper torso plane. In other words, the legs remain within the parameters of the upper torso. Also, the posture exhibits tensegrity by adjusting to change with minimal energy usage, yet still providing a strong structure.

The Yijikim Yeungma is particularly suitable for women because a woman has a wider pelvis than a man, and her pelvis-femur joints are farther apart than are a man's. In order to minimize the stress on the back and knees, especially during pregnancy, the female's femur bones veer towards the center at the knees. If they went straight down vertically from the pelvis-femur joints like men's do, their legs (particularly their knees) would be farther away from the line of gravity where the fetus would be carried, which would impart stress to the knees and back. The inward-pointing femur at the knees will give them a "spring" with which to absorb the shock when walking and carrying a child.

So, by design, women ride the Yijikim Yeungma horse on a daily basis. Most women can comfortably bring their knees together when they lower themselves in the Yijikim Yeungma position, whereas men have difficulty doing this without forcibly squeezing their knees inward. When you squeeze your knees inward, you are taxing your muscles and burning energy, so it will defeat the purpose of having a strong and low-energy consuming structure. However, if you can do it comfortably, it will form an even stronger structure than when the knees are open. By closing the gap at the knees, you will form a true triangle with your lower legs and the ground. You will lower your center of gravity to the knees, and, thus, will be able to resist upper and frontal forces from that point, since the apex of a triangle is its strongest point.

Another thing to note about the Yijikim Yeungma posture relative to the theory of tensegrity is that we're held together by soft tissues and tendons pulling the muscles (and thus the bones) from the top to the sacrum, and pulling from the bottom to the sacrum, just like all the spokes of a bicycle wheel merging towards the hub. So, if we were to relax some of the muscles, soft tissues, and tendons holding the lower trunk up, our legs will lower our structure; and if our heels were turned outward in the Yijikim Yeungma position, we would then drop down on our knees—not to the ground, but knee to knee. What this means is that when you relax your tendons and leg muscles, you will naturally fall into the Yijikim Yeungma position, provided that your bone structure was designed that way. Relaxation is one of the key components of martial arts. Relaxation, not to the point of being lethargic or asleep, but rather making use of the minimum amount of tendons and muscles required to execute a particular movement. This is achieved by not taxing any leg muscles and tendons that will siphon away the energy of other muscles and tendons.

Our tendons and muscles are always in a tensed position to hold us up. However, this tension should be like the fan belt in your car; if you make it any tighter than it needs to be, it will stress the tendons/belt, and if you make it any looser than it has to be, it will cause a lag in reaction. Therefore, when you let the tendons and muscles of your legs sit in a perfectly tensed position that is not struggling against gravity, your legs will be most stable (for balance), efficient (for reaction) and strong (for delivering force).

The Wing Chun developers must have experimented and learned of the benefits of the Yijikim Yeungma posture and incorporated it into the Wing Chun system. Even if Abbess Ng Mui and Yim Wing Chun did not take the Yijikim Yeungma posture from the mountain girls of Yunnan, or invent the Yijikim Yeungma, then Doctor Leung Jan would have done it anyway. He was a Chinese physician. Every Chinese physician was (and still is) an anatomist.

THE WARHORSE

As is the case with most Asian martial arts, one of the cardinal principles in Wing Chun is to maintain stability. Every form in Wing Chun usually begins with a movement that pertains to the stance or warhorse. The pelvis and waist area is where the main engine resides to control the horse and deliver force to both the horse and its rider. There is little to any focus on the shoulders in the Wing Chun stance as this power structure forms a triangle, with the shoulders representing the pinnacle point of the triangle, the legs representing the base, and the waist in between. In contrast, the typical image in the West of a strong man is that of a person who has broad shoulders, a narrow waist and light-footed legs, forming an inverted triangle. Most Western sports involve running and, therefore, like a racehorse, having light legs are advantageous in such sports.

Structurally, however, there is a trade off between stability and mobility. When a structure is designed for stability, there is less mobility; and conversely, when a structure is designed for mobility, there is less stability. In other words, the more stability you want, the less mobility you will have and the more mobility you want, the less stability you will have.

So in designing a martial art, one has to decide which is the more important attribute. Many people believe that the ideal would be a 50–50 compromise. However, that is comparable to sitting on a fence, unable to decide one way or another. In fact, being a perfect compromise, you would end up being perfectly compromised—being neither strongly grounded nor swiftly mobile. Remember, we have an S-shaped spine and a tension system that allows us to walk, run, sit, lie down, bend, and perform other tasks that do not require exceptional stability or mobility skills. However, when exceptional stability or mobility is required, we require special training to condition our bodies to produce them. A sprinter requires specific training to become a better sprinter; a marathon runner requires specific training in order to successfully run a marathon; a swimmer requires specific training to improve as a swimmer; an acrobat requires specific training to become a better acrobat, and a boxer requires specific training to become a better boxer. And so it goes with every skill set that we wish to develop. The mind and body must both be trained for each and every specific task we wish to improve in. It is another example of the Specific Adaptation to Imposed Demands Principle (S.A.I.D.) mentioned earlier.

Let's examine the sport of boxing for a moment. The concept underpinning boxing is for the boxer to become very mobile, thus enabling the boxer to dodge, twist, bend, skip, sprint, and dance out of harm's way. Therefore a boxer needs his upper torso and lower trunk to be both mobile and agile. However, he also needs to be grounded if he wishes to deliver a powerful punch—but he doesn't need to be grounded at all times. He only needs to be grounded when the opportunity to deliver a telling blow presents itself. In boxing the athlete is only allowed to punch above his opponent's waist using the front of his gloves; tripping, sweeping, throwing, kicking, elbowing, grappling, head-butting, kneeing, choking, and a whole slew of other street-fighting tactics are not allowed in this sport. So, when none of these are of concern, stability is of little importance. The only arsenal he and his opponent have are gloved fists. Therefore, he can bounce on his toes, stop to hit, and go back to bouncing. His life is not being threatened; he doesn't need to immobilize, maim, or kill his opponent; he just needs to knock him out, TKO him, or rack up more points than his opponent within the twelve rounds that are available to him to do this.

By contrast, Wing Chun wasn't designed for sport. It was designed for personal protection—the kind of situations where one might find one's life at risk. The goals, principles and strategies, therefore, are entirely different from those used in sport of any kind. Stability in Wing Chun is of utmost importance. For this reason, Wing Chun's strategy is to not kick from a distance, but to kick from close range when one has one's upper body already in contact with his opponent's. The Wing Chun practitioner will use this contact to stabilize himself. Other than in the Yijikim Yeungma position, a properly-trained Wing Chun practitioner is poised to put his weight on his rear leg and heel. It can be 90–10, 80–20, 70–30, 60–40, or even 55–45—but never 50–50. The rear leg is always the root, and the front is the stabilizer. The reason for this is once you lift the front leg to kick (or use your rear leg to kick—which would then make the front leg become the rear and rooted leg), you lose your stabilizer. However, when you have some kind of contact with your opponent with your arm or arms, his grounded legs become your stabilizer.

Stability is very important in Wing Chun's fighting concept and training; however, that doesn't mean that the practitioner is going to remain static throughout a fight. It just means that the practitioner should not move, and particularly not retreat, unnecessarily. Typically, most martial artists, including Wing Chun practitioners, and just about every person without formal martial arts training, will take a step backwards when an opponent takes a step forward. They just like to keep that comfortable and non-threatening distance between them. As a result, there is nothing gained from such a move by either of them, except that they've just moved to a different position. If anything, it would be disadvantageous for the one who retreats because he doesn't have eyes in the back of his head, and could step somewhere (or into) something harmful. Also running backward will always be slower and more difficult than running forward; therefore, the advancing attacker will eventually catch up to the backward runner, and possible make the backward runner fall.

If an attacker rushed forward with an attack, and you stepped back out of harm's way, you would probably be out of range to strike him as well, which takes your offensive weapons (your ability to end a fight) out of play. Even if you were able to hit him somehow while in retreat, it would not be a very powerful blow, and certainly not powerful enough to cause much damage because your body would be traveling backward while your fist was traveling forward. In other words, the backward motion would negate the power of the forward strike. It would be like trying to hit a long drive in golf by hurling yourself backward while swinging your golf club forward.

The fighting stance (or warhorse) in Wing Chun must therefore be strong and stable; it must be up to withstanding incoming force. By the same token, however, it must have the strength to advance and bridge the distance between you and your opponent, or to ram the opponent's horse, kick it, break its legs, or knock and trample the rider and horse down. This is achieved through the progressive training contained in Wing Chun's six forms and the drills that accompany them.

Learning martial art is learning the properties of force; thus enabling us to utilize our bodies to generate the maximum amount of force, whether it is of the compression or tension type, or differentiating and understanding the relationship between kinetic and potential energy, so that, ultimately, we learn how to produce maximum results from a minimum of effort.

Returning to the topic of weight differential in regards to stance, I would like to attempt to quell the ongoing argument amongst Wing Chun practitioners as to whether one should distribute one's weight evenly on both legs (50–50) or whether the weight should rest predominantly on the rear leg when one leg is in front of the other.

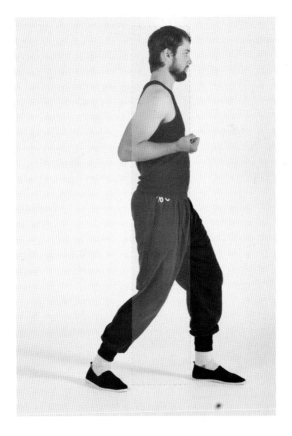

Jingseung Ma (Front-Body Horse) with 50–50 weight distribution

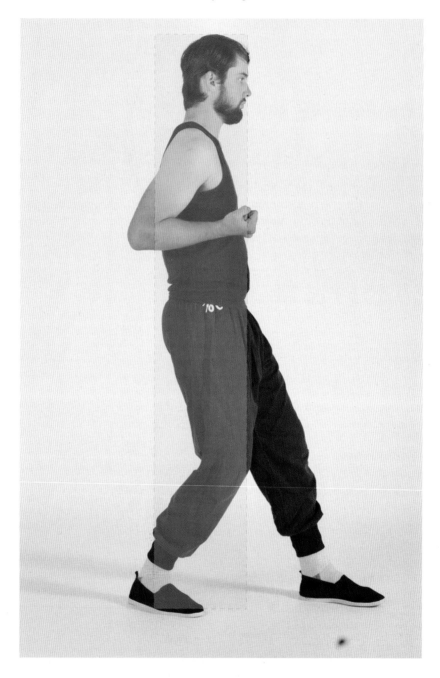

Jingseung Ma (Front-Body Horse) with upper torso weight predominantly over rear leg

THE TAO OF WALKING

Let's first look at how we use two different classes of energy to walk. From a square and frontal natural stance, when a person takes his first step to walk, he might push off with his right leg as if a pendulum has been nudged. As he pushes off with his right leg his torso leans forward and lets his left leg fall forward. In this instant he has used his stored potential energy to shove himself off. This potential energy is then transferred to kinetic energy as the opposite leg begins to "fall" toward the ground.

When that foot lands on the ground, he's at the end of the pendulum arc, at which point the pendulum's velocity and kinetic energy are at its maximum. If he were to continue this pendulum effect, he would then use his left foot and ankle to shove off (like a pole-vault), continuing from the bottom of the arc to the top of the opposite high-end of the arc, at which point he would be standing with 100 percent of his weight on his left leg, and preparing to move his upper body and right leg forward for the next pendulum swing. He would now be at a point where the kinetic energy is at its minimum, but the potential energy (i.e., mass x gravity x height) is at its peak. When his whole structure, from top to bottom, is aligned to the Line of Gravity, especially when in motion, he will have the greatest potential energy. When he steps forward and in midst of a complete cycle; i.e., when his upper torso is centered between his legs, with a weight distribution of 50–50, he has maximum kinetic energy. However, if he doesn't use the maximum kinetic energy to move forward, he will have "maxed out" this energy.

If I hold a pendulum at either high-end of the arc, it will always have maximum potential energy. It will transfer to kinetic energy only when I release it. The pendulum will reach its maximum kinetic force at the bottom of the arc, at which point it will begin to diminish. When it reaches the top of the other end of the arc, it will transfer to maximum potential energy. However, if I stop or hold the pendulum and let it rest at the bottom end of the arc, it will have diminished both the potential and kinetic energy. It will then require extra energy to move the pendulum up to the top of the arc, to begin the process anew.

Understanding this, when it comes to the issue of a fighting stance, you can better appreciate why resting one's upper torso between one's widespread legs in a stationary position is no different than being at the bottom of the pendulum arc or pendulum at rest. Such a posture just doesn't allow for any mobility as a lot of people claim. It is only good if you continue walking, but not planting yourself for a stationary position. When walking, you will spend the least amount of time in this position.

Whereas, there is a millisecond pause (as with a pendulum) when you are in the upright feet-together position, which serves as the highest point of a pendulum's swinging arc. If you watch a slow-motion video of someone walking, you will see that the person will be on the one leg upright position two to three times as long as when he has both feet on the ground in the 50-50 position. In other words, the 50–50 weight-distribution posture does not allow efficient mobility as claimed by its proponents. It is only good as an interim phase between movements. This is why practitioners who use this posture can be seen subconsciously rocking themselves back and forth before the actual engagement with an opponent—at which time they try to stabilize themselves, but seldom are they able to do so successfully.

When pressure is applied against a person in this position from the front, back, or side, he will not have any strength to resist it because neither side of the upper sagittal torso is directly supported by either of his legs. His posture or structure has no weight bearing strength, and therefore, no foundation or resisting strength.

Unlike a natural frontal standing position of 50–50 weight distribution where each side of the upper torso is directly supported by each leg, the 50–50 weight distribution posture of one leg placed in front of the other with the upper torso suspended between the legs is unstable, structurally weak and consumes a needlessly high amount of energy to sustain. By nature, living beings do things with the least amount of energy if possible. For this reason, we never stand with one foot in front of the other (with the upper torso suspended in between) when we wait for a bus, stand with the crowd in an open air concert, or stand and chat with a friend in the street. Instead, we assume a natural standing posture. If we get tired or stiff, we shift to one leg or the other, but we never assume a 50–50 weight distribution with one leg in front of the other.

From the day we first learned to stand and walk we were abiding by the principles of physics and human anatomy. At such a young age we were not conscious of these principles, but they were in effect nonetheless as we learned to successfully navigate around our surroundings. Over the years and decades our minds learned how to make better application of these principles by taking advantage of the mechanics of standing, walking, and running. Although we may not have learned to do them as efficiently as possible, nor as efficiently as some other people, we nevertheless learned to do them well enough to employ these principles for the rest of our lives. However, if we can find a way to improve our understanding and application of these principles, it will only yield us a greater benefit—so why not do it? Similarly, in Wing Chun, we must continue to look for ways to discover the most economical, efficient and effective way of doing things. And we can only do that by better understanding biomechanics and the laws of physics that relate to them.

Wing Chun practitioners that advocate the even-weight distribution like to argue that the 50–50 weight distribution gives them more mobility, but never have any explanations as to why—either scientifically or hypothetically. That's the way they answer all the intelligent questions a student asks. When a student asks, "Why do we punch this way?" or "Why do we block this way?" The answers come back, "Because it is stronger and faster!" or "It is more economical, efficient, and effective!" Well, we can say that about everything, but tell me exactly "why?" and "how?" Does any fighting system intentionally teach uneconomical, inefficient and ineffective ways of doing things? Don't they also believe that their ways are the best? So, if you are going to convince your student as to why and how your system is superior, shouldn't you at least be giving him or her some in-depth and scientifically valid answers?

Beside its weakness in the static position, the 50–50 distribution stance is also impractical in combat. In order to advance or retreat, the practitioner must first bring his upper torso to the front leg before he can safely stabilize and move his rear leg forward, or move his torso back to his rear leg to stabilize before he can move his front leg back. In other words, he needs to stabilize first before he can act on anything, whether to walk, punch or kick. Whether he kicks with his front leg or rear leg, he will need to shift his weight forward or backward first before he can do it; and this will be slower, more energy consuming and less efficient. Also, when he lifts his front foot to step forward, his upper torso will have lost its support. Each leg in the 50–50 position only served to brace his upper torso angularly against gravity's perpendicular force; the two legs, in essence, were pressing against each other to hold the upper torso upright. Once he lifts one of those legs, he will no longer have any brace to hold him up. If he lifts his front foot, then the force of gravity will pull him down to the front. The only recourse left for him is to put that foot down again quickly to prevent him from falling. However, a smart opponent could prevent that by sweeping his leg before it lands.

If a 50–50 braced structure were more efficient and effective against gravity and other natural forces, then all lampposts, buildings, and other vertical structures would have been designed with two angular posts under them instead of planting these structures directly in the ground in line with the Line of Gravity. Chairs and tables would have legs that angled out as well. If they were designed that way, their joints would constantly be under stress, and eventually would be brought down by the force of gravity.

[111]

Now, before we look into the benefits of Wing Chun's rear-weighted horse stance, let's examine another favored horse stance in the martial arts community, the Bow-and-Arrow stance.

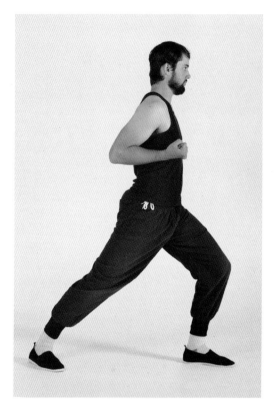

The classic Bow-and-Arrow
stance of other martial arts

The Bow-and-Arrow stance has the martial artist place his upper torso towards his front leg by bending his front leg to a position near 90 degrees, while his rear leg is stretched and straight. This serves to lower his Center of Gravity (CoG) as well as widen the base of his structure. Although lowering the Center of Gravity will somewhat stabilize his balance, he will find that he is unable to position his upper torso directly over his front leg. The front leg will always be ahead of his torso; therefore, it is still not aligned to the perpendicular Line of Gravity, and therefore, he is not optimally balanced.

The other problem with the Bow-and-Arrow stance is that the front knee is put under a lot of strain. Any knee bent at 90 degrees or near this position will stress and possibly damage the ligaments, tendons, and muscles if performed regularly and over extended periods of time. As far as potential energy is concerned, this stance has nearly "zero" value for any movement going forward. It will require a lot of effort to raise the front knee as the rear leg has already exhausted all of its potential energy from being in a straightened position. It will have a higher value for retreating backward when the front leg is used to shove the upper torso backward and if the rear knee is allowed to bend. So, as far as mobility is concerned, it has very little value.

Although this stance will provide strong resistance against a pressure that is applied from the front (because the rear leg is braced angularly towards the force), it will only have "resistant" force. It simply does not have any potential energy or mechanism to push the structure forward; both the legs in this posture have exhausted the potential energy and leverage completely.

If someone were to pull you while you were in this stance, you would have very little strength and leverage to resist the pull because of the stance being more lead-foot loaded. You would need to change your posture so that your rear leg is bent and your front leg is straightened before you could generate any strength or leverage.

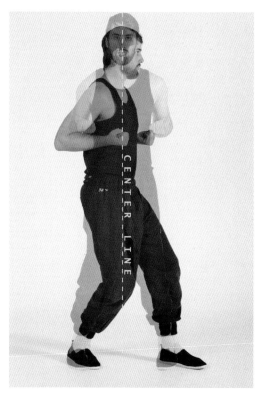

Yijikim Yeungma rotated 45 degrees becomes Jingseung Ma (JSM).

Now let's look at Wing Chun's rear-weighted horse stance. It is actually just the Yijikim Yeungma turned 45 degrees to the side. If you don't believe me, try it: stand in the Yijikim Yeungma position in front of a full-length mirror and make a note of where your Centerline is in reference to the background or a marking on the mirror. If you don't have a long mirror, just draw a line on the floor to mark your Centerline between your feet. Now, slowly rotate your pelvis, shoulders and feet (with fixed heels) to your left, around the Centerline. Make sure by cross-referencing the Centerline mark with your Centerline. When you've turned about 45 degrees, look at where your upper torso is in relation to your legs. You will see that your torso and Centerline are now closer to the rear leg instead of the 50–50 position that you began with in Yijikim Yeungma. In order for you to distribute your upper torso weight 50–50 onto each leg, you will need to move the Centerline, thus the upper torso, forward. If you have previously practiced Wing Chun's second form, Chum Kiu (尋橋—Seeking the Bridge), you may not have noticed this phenomenon because you were habitually moving your Centerline back and forth during the Chum Kiu rotation. In Chum Kiu's first section, you rotate 180 degrees from left to right and from right to left. If you rotate around your Centerline, you will surely end up sitting on your rear leg. However, if you try to distribute the weight of your upper torso evenly on both legs, you will end up "shifting" the Centerline back and forth—which is more energy-consuming and less stable. On the other hand, if you rotate around your Centerline, you will expend a lot less energy and not compromise your balance by uprooting and moving your Centerline (which also is your line of gravity) every time you rotate.

This demonstrates that the most efficient way of rotating your structure is to maintain your Centerline and rotate one whole sagittal side and leg into the Centerline. Shifting the Centerline from one position to another is energy consuming, slow and unstable. This happens not only when practitioners adjust themselves to the 50–50 position, but also to those who spin on the balls or the middle of their feet, as well as those who lean back too much on their rear leg.

From the Yijikim Yeungma position, you can't help but rotate from the middle because you are standing at a 50–50 weight-distributed position. However, once the turn is complete, and your body is twisted (as opposed to being squared where the shoulder plane is vertically aligned to pelvis plane), you would naturally assume the rear-weighed position (as just explained). From here, it would be more efficient to rotate the pelvis from the side where your upper body is aligned with the weight-bearing leg. In other words, you will rotate the side that has a full vertical shaft that is perpendicularly grounded. This would be much more efficient than using an angled fulcrum or an invisible one. You can't call an imaginary perpendicular line below your coccyx and between your feet a fulcrum (as the 50–50 advocates believe). An invisible fulcrum is no fulcrum at all. A fulcrum must be fixed and grounded—it can't be imaginary or mobile. Although your spine, which is attached to your pelvis and is grounded by your 50–50 weight distribution on your legs, can act as a fulcrum, it can only be a fulcrum to your upper body. When rotating just the upper body, you will shear and weaken your structure. To truly rotate your structure efficiently and effectively, one sagittal side (upper and lower torso) must be fixed perpendicularly to the ground, and is used to power the rotation of the free sagittal side. This is not dissimilar to how a door works. A door is hinged to a vertical frame, which is fixed to a firmly grounded wall, allowing it to swing freely without causing stress to the hinges from gravity or human force.

I am often asked which side of the pelvis should be used to rotate the structure—the front-leg side or the rear-leg side? Let's reword the question for more clarity. Which pelvic and hip muscles should you use to initiate the rotation—the ones from the free sagittal side or the ones from the grounded side? For the 50–50 advocates, it makes no difference because both sides have equal properties. For that matter, in that position, their femurs (thigh bones) are in the middle of the hip-joint sockets and are not pressured enough by the upper torso to lock it in position to rotate it in real time. When either side of the pelvic and hip-joint muscles are called upon to rotate the pelvis, the upper torso rotates first, almost 90 degrees before locking the joint, whereupon another set of muscles are called upon to rotate the femur. In other words, there is poor coordination and lag between the rotation of the upper torso and lower trunk and the muscles that are involved. By contrast, those weighing their upper torsos predominantly on their rear legs have their femurs nearly locked into the hip-joint socket, allowing them to use the rear sagittal side's pelvic and hip muscles to turn the upper torso no more than 45 degrees to put it in the fully locked position and rotate the femur with little or no help from its muscles. Using one set of muscles predominantly, rotating on a vertical and grounded fulcrum, rotating around the Centerline (which is also the Line of Gravity and fulcrum) in a small arc, and not changing fulcrums midstream, makes the rotation economical, efficient, and powerful. In the full 180-degree rotation that you perform in the Chum Kiu form, you would transfer the force of the rotation from one sagittal side to the other exactly at the point when the femur locks into the hip joint. At this time, you will free the original grounded sagittal side to become the free-swinging side. The action would be like you pushing hard on a door to open it but someone resists it from the other side and then suddenly releases his force—the door would then swing open forcefully.

If the above explanation doesn't do it for the 50–50 advocates or the free-side initiators, then here are some more examples as to why the rear-weighted posture is more beneficial than the 50–50 posture.

Hold a geometric compass by its head, plant the arm with the metal tip to a piece of paper, and use it as the fulcrum, then draw a circle with the pencil tip. Notice that you will need to move your hand and arm in a complete circle to draw the penciled circle.

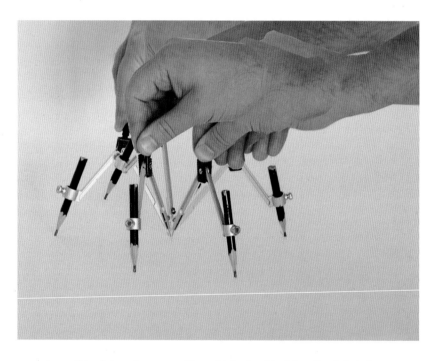

An equilateral-shaped compass will require the hand to follow the circle it draws.

Now, adjust the compass so that the penciled arm is long enough to make the metal-tip arm nearly perpendicular to the paper. Draw a circle now, and notice how you only need to twirl your thumb and finger in one stationary position—rather than your entire hand and arm—to accomplish the job.

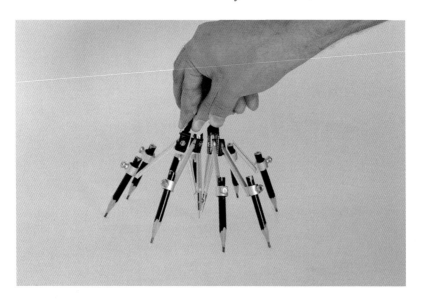

With a right-triangle-shaped compass, the hand remains nearly stationary, using only the thumb and index fingers to twirl the fulcrum and draw a circle.

By performing these two experiments you will see firsthand how economical and efficient it is to rotate the penciled arm of the compass when the fulcrum is perpendicular; whereas, when the fulcrum is angled, it will require more energy and movement.

When you ride a horse bareback, like how the Native Americans did—without the saddle, headstall, and accessories—you sit upright and control the turns using your lower trunk (pelvis, hip, and thighs). A good motorcyclist does the same. He doesn't turn the handlebars nor lean with his head and shoulders. A cavalier needs his hands to wield his weapons; thus, control the horse with his lower trunk instead of the reins. He must keep his upper torso upright to maintain balance; he cannot swing it to rotate his horse.

If by some chance you become a cavalier (or a quartermaster for the ancient army), you must select a horse suitable for warfare. You must consider its breed (type), structure, strength, balance, and mental state. When the horse meets your criteria, you select it. However, that wouldn't be the end of the task. The horse is untrained, and so are you. You will need to train yourselves to become one with the horse and the horse to become one with you. The horse will need to train for battle, and maintain its structure, balance, and strength under all circumstances. You will need to train

yourself to stay mounted and command the horse correctly under all circumstances. When you battle a mounted opponent, your horse will also battle his horse. The breed of horse that the Wing Chun founders selected for
their fighting system was the Yijikim Yeungma—a very strong and capable
horse that can easily adapt to changes.

A rider of the Yijikim Yeungma just needs the one horse for all battle situations. He doesn't need to change horses like riders in other armies.
Whether he faces the opponent from the front or sideways (or even with his
back to him), he can easily change angles. He doesn't need to change to a
Front-Facing Horse, a Back-Sitting Horse, a Side-Riding Horse, a Crouching
Tiger, a Cat Stance, a Crane Pose, or any other animal posture; he can adapt
to the situation by merely turning himself or his horse.

When I learned Wing Chun in the seventies, there was never any talk
of the Jingseung Ma (Front-Body Horse or Front-Facing Horse)—正身馬 or
Pian Seung Ma (Side-Body Horse or Side-Facing Horse)—偏身馬. It was just
the Yijikim Yeungma—because that was all there was.

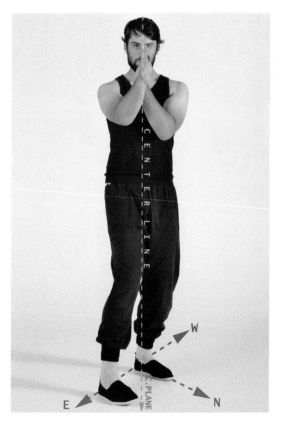

Jingseung Ma—Front-Body
Horse

[118]

Suppose you were in the Yijikim Yeungma posture facing north with your right Wusau (護手—Guarding Hand) in front of the left in the en-garde position, and your opponent was positioned northeast—and you turned your structure towards him (hands pointing at his Centerline). Your thigh would meet the Line of Gravity/Centerline, as long as you maintained the Line of Gravity in its original Yijikim Yeungma position and rotated around it. This will put you in a rear-weighted position with one leg in front of the other—the Jingseung Ma (Front-Body Horse) position—in relation to him.

Now, if you were facing north, and your opponent was right in front of you, and you had your right Wusau in front of the left in the en-garde position pointing at his Centerline—and you turned just your horse (lower trunk) northwest (45 degrees), you'd have the Pian Seung Ma (Side-Body Horse) in relation to him. It's as simple as that!

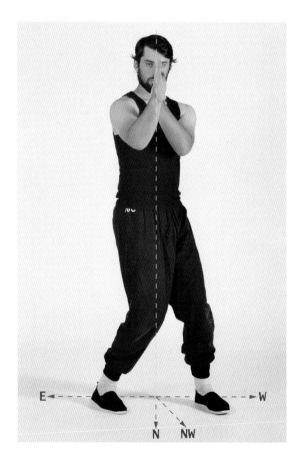

Pian Seung Ma—Side-Body Horse

[119]

Yijikim Yeungma has many faces; all that Jingseung Ma and Pian Seung Ma represent is the Yijikim Yeungma at different angles. The Wing Chun System makes this very easy by starting all of its forms with the Yijikim Yeungma position, then changing the angle of the horse within the forms, but always returning back to the square Yijikim Yeungma position. The rider and the horse (upper and lower torso) will always share and use the same Centerline, Line of Gravity, and fulcrum, although the two may face different directions.

Although you could rotate your horse 90 degrees from the square Yijikim Yeungma position (from facing north to facing east), it would be a position (still a Jingseung Ma) that you'd want to avoid when facing your opponent. In that position, both of your feet would be on the Centerline Plane that extends from your Centerline to your opponent's Centerline. This would be analogous to standing on a tight rope; your balance would be vulnerable to falling to the sides. In this position, you would be standing sideways in relation to your opponent, allowing him to kick the side of your knee, topple you, or step to your side easily.

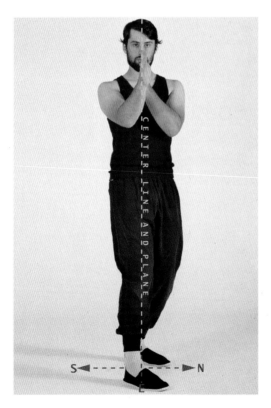

Your balance is vulnerable when both feet are standing on the Centerline Plane, or both heels are on the same plane.

[120]

At this point, some Wing Chun practitioners might argue that in the first section of the Chum Kiu (Seeking the Bridge) form we begin from the Yijikim Yeungma position and then rotate 90 degrees, and then 180 degrees to the other side and then back again, which makes us stand on one line. And then in Sections Two and Three, we walk on one line one way, turn around, and walk back on the same line. Why?

When you think of the movements in the forms strictly as techniques and applications—like many Wing Chun practitioners do—then many movements within the forms do not make sense. This is why practitioners often perform their forms mindlessly; they simply don't understand why and what they are doing. As a result, they cannot transfer the movements from the forms into sparring or fighting situations. As mentioned earlier, the forms are nothing more than secret user manuals that contain the principles of Wing Chun, information on the tools of Wing Chun, instructions on how to use these tools in conjunction with the principles, and exercises that develop the mind and body for the Wing Chun system, along with some examples for application. They were designed to intentionally throw off those who were trying to learn the secrets of the art through casual observation.

When you understand the true purpose of the forms, then you will understand why the forms require you to do things that don't quite seem to add up.

In reality, when sparring or fighting, you will never rotate your structure 180 degrees from east to west. The most you would rotate is 90 degrees. The opponent will almost always be in front of you. Wherever he moves, you will always line your sight and Centerline to his Centerline—and this goes for all fighters, not just Wing Chun practitioners. No one is going to allow the opponent to come around to one's side or back if he can help it. He will always turn to face the opponent.

In the Chum Kiu form, you are learning how to rotate your structure powerfully. You will use this rotation to torque your structure and deliver its force onto wherever you make contact with your opponent, whether it be a strike, a push, or a pull. When your opponent is in front of you, the most that you can rotate (and all that you require) is 45 degrees of rotation from the Yijikim Yeungma square position, and 90 degrees from the Pian Seung Ma or Jingseung Ma position. The 180-degree rotation seen in the Chum Kiu form is not for you to rotate from north to south to strike an opponent behind you with a Lansau (攔手—Barring Arm) or Mansau (問手—Probing Arm) as demonstrated by some sifus. That kind of explanation can be expected from a beginner or a spectator with no martial arts experience, but coming from a sifu it is rather disappointing. As long as you don't

[121]

have eyes in the back of your head, you wouldn't know if an opponent was behind you or how far away he was from you to confidently turn around and hit him accurately. This type of sifu glories in fighting multiple opponents that he has placed just where he wants them to be, and they attack him just when and in the manner that he wants them to. He will demonstrate how he can knock down the first attacker, and he'll turn around to knock down the opponent behind him, and then the opponents on his side one-by-one. Well, what makes him so sure that he'd knock the first opponent down with just one move? In reality, if he didn't knock out the first opponent, the others would be all over him simultaneously.

I had a good laugh with a video clip on YouTube, where an American Wing Chun master went against a Russian wrestler in a cage fight. Before the fight, the TV broadcaster showed a demonstration of the Wing Chun guy surrounded by five or six of his students. In they came and he knocked out each student with just one blow each within seconds. The commentators were saying how difficult it would be for the wrestler to fight someone like him. However, when the two got inside the ring, the wrestler choked the Wing Chun master out within seconds. It's best never to focus too much on scenarios where you'll be fighting multiple assailants; it is difficult enough to fight just one person who is standing right in front of you.

Allow me a minute to explain why the Chum Kiu form makes the student rotate 180 degrees and also walk on one line. In all Wing Chun forms, you learn to develop good habits and learn about your parameters. You learn how far your strike can reach in the square and angled positions; you learn how far you can push or pull; you learn how far, near, high, low, and sideways you can place your limbs in relation to your body; and you learn how soft, firm, slow, and fast you can move your limbs and body. What you are doing here is learning to expand your range.

In the Chum Kiu form, although you are least likely to rotate a full 180 degrees on one line in a real fight, the training from this form will take you to the extreme that you can turn in order to maximize your power and balance. When you get to the point where you can rotate 180 degrees with both power and stability, it will help you to be able to rotate to a 45-degree angle with more power and more stability.

In the Wing Chun training program, we're learning to deal with situations where the opponent has an upper hand momentarily. This is the reality of warfare. We must experience these positions in training so that we can react accordingly when in actual combat. We must experience both our limitations and capabilities to fully understand them. This is why we put ourselves in such situations. Standing on a narrow surface is a situation that you will often encounter in training, but you should not consciously place yourself at such a disadvantage during a fight. Nevertheless, by training this position you can learn what you must do to survive and escape if you ever find yourself in such a position.

While we must learn to recover from a vulnerable situation, we must also learn to develop good habits that will not cause us to find ourselves in such circumstances. So, Wing Chun's training program isn't always about putting you in such situations, but rather to train you to develop good sense, good posture, and good balance.

As for the apparent step-sliding on one line in Sections Two and Three of the Chum Kiu form, you actually aren't doing that. In Section Two, you don't do the Gwansau (滚手—Rolling Arms) in the direction of the walk, but actually at an angle that is 90 degrees from it. That is, if you started the form facing north in the Yijikim Yeungma posture, and performed the first movement of rotating and kicking west, followed by landing the foot on the east-west line, you would do the Gwansau movement towards the north. So, in reference to the opponent, you wouldn't be standing on his or your Centerline Plane. Your Gwansau will go one direction, and your horse will go in another. You are in effect in the Pian Seung Ma position relative to him. (I'll explain a little later as to why this is done that way.)

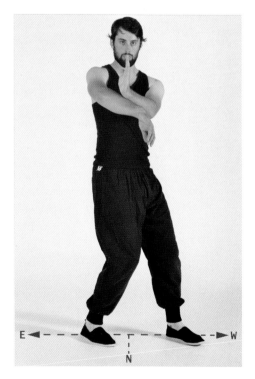

Gwansau (Rolling Arms) is directed northward, while the horse charges westward.

[123]

In Section Three, you don't walk on one line either. After you execute your first left kick, you don't land your heel on the same line as the right, but land it a bit to the left of it, and left of the Centerline Plane. This way, you have the Centerline between your heels. In this position, your heels are on two lines, giving you the stability you need, and yet protecting your groin with your knees. Also, after step-sliding three times, you take a half step to join the right foot with the left side-by-side. If the left foot wasn't on a separate line, you couldn't do it properly. It will be in the way of the right foot or you will need to adjust your feet and body positions to somehow compensate the awkwardness.

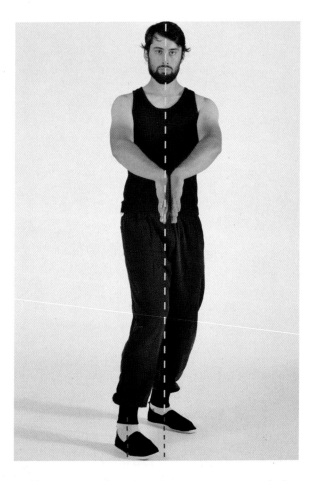

Double Bongsau performed on the Jingseung Ma; rear heel is aligned with the front toes.

I have a theory that the original Chum Kiu form may not have been a linear walking form, but that it was converted to a linear form after it came to the Wing Chun practitioners in the Red Junk Operas.

For all practical purposes, you wouldn't rotate your structure more than 45 degrees. Once you rotate more than that, you will expose your back to your opponent and make yourself extremely vulnerable to attacks from the side, the back and, of course, to takedowns. I believe that the original Section-I of the Chum Kiu form may have had the practitioner rotate only 45 degrees on the first rotation, and 90 degrees on the next two; for Section II, it may have had the practitioner kick and walk 45 degrees from the original Yijikim Yeungma northern position towards the northwest, and then walk northeast for the second half. In Section III, the practitioner would again kick and walk 45 degrees towards the northwest, followed by walking 45 degrees northeast. In other words, the practitioner would have advanced northward in a zigzag pattern. It all makes sense because in this way you would always be facing your opponent rather than changing the position of the opponent from one place to another throughout the form.

With that in mind, using the Gwansau movement in Section II begins to make sense. When an opponent (positioned in the north) strikes you with his left hand from the front, there is no reason why you'd Gwansau (right Bongsau—膀手 Wing Arm—and left Wusau—護手 Guard Hand) and walk eastward. If you did, you might be able to deflect his left-hand strike, but you would walk right into his following right-hand strike. However, if you Gwan (滾 rolled) his strike and walk towards him at a 45 degree angle, your Gwansau—now strongly supported by your Pian Seung Ma (Side-Body Horse)—will disrupt his balance and disable any forthcoming attack.

Why do you think the founders of Wing Chun changed the 45-degree walk to linear in Chum Kiu and Biu Jee? For one, they may have done it to conceal the truth. Second, the Red Junk practitioners may have done it because of the lack of space on their boats. The zigzag pattern would have taken up a lot more space—particularly if two or more practitioners trained together.

One important thing to know about the Jingseung Ma position of the Yijikim Yeungma structure is that the rear sagittal side must be firmly grounded while the front sagittal side must be mobile. Like a door, as long as the door is free-swinging, it will not put stress on the frame or the wall. If the hinges were not free swinging and were stiff instead, a strong swing of the door could tear the hinge or frame off the wall. This is why you want a solid structure and fulcrum, but a free-swinging door. Similarly, you want your front sagittal side to swing freely from your rear and vertically planted side. This would be hard to accomplish for the 50–50 weighted and front-foot weighted practitioners. For the 50–50 practitioners, without a vertical or dominant fulcrum, the whole structure would be susceptible for a teardown. For the front-foot weighted practitioners, they are offering a fulcrum and grounded side well within the reach of the opponent. A small force towards this fulcrum by an opponent will turn your whole structure around in just the same way that a small twirl on the head of a compass will rotate both of its arms in a circle.

When you put your weight on your front leg and use your back leg as the stabilizer, your front leg becomes the fulcrum. What's the problem with this? For one thing, you've lost a "backing" force, just as if you stood right beside a desk instead of behind it to push it. If you have one foot in front of the other—whether you punch with your left or right arm, the power comes from the rear leg. Here's a quick experiment:

Stand approximately two feet away from a wall with your left foot in front of your right, and press your right fist against the wall at roughly the height of your solar plexus. Now push your fist hard into the wall and, while sustaining this pressure, lift your left foot up. No problem, right? Next, repeat the process but this time attempt to lift your right leg up. It doesn't happen, does it? Why, because the force is always delivered and countered by your rear leg. Now if do the same experiment with the same leg positions but using the alternate fist; i.e., pressing into the wall with your left fist this time, you will now have your left leg and hand in front, and your right leg still behind. Again, without releasing the pressure of your left fist on the wall, lift your front foot. No problem. Next, without releasing the arm pressure, lift your rear leg. You still can't do it! You can even begin by lifting the heel up from the rear foot and go on your toes (as in the Jeet Kune Do On-Guard Stance) with this experiment and you still won't be able to lift the rear foot without releasing the pressure of the arm and having to lean even closer. So, it goes without saying that the less weight you have on your rear leg, the less support you will get from it, and the less force you will deliver.

That is not to say that it is totally impossible to deliver *any* force when you are front-foot weighted. After all, Bruce Lee used the front side as the fulcrum to rotate the front of his pelvis to torque his lead punch and he was able to generate plenty of power! Boxers have been doing this for ages as well with their lead hook punches. What I'm saying is that you will deliver *more* power by rotating from the back. If you want every punch to be a knockout, it is best to keep your rear foot grounded.

The other problem with a lead leg–weighted stance, as I mentioned earlier, is that with such a stance your fulcrum would be within the reach of your opponent. A rear fulcrum would be like the axle of a wheel; in this case, we'll look at the wheel as if it were in a horizontal position. If you hand the axle to a person, he can turn it (thus turning the whole wheel) or take it anywhere he wants. Whereas, if you keep it out of his reach, and put a rim around it, he can only turn the rim (which requires much more effort—like the grinders in an ancient mill), and will not affect the axle.

When you are on your front leg predominantly, your balance will be susceptible and you won't be able to generate maximum power. Wrestlers poise themselves in a crouching position for this reason; they have both of their legs behind their upper torsos so that they can generate more pushing power, and prevent their opponents from grabbing their legs and toppling them down. Because they don't put any emphasis on slugging, they don't need to be upright and/or have one leg in front of the other for torque power. Wrestlers use mostly compression and tension forces rather than kinetic force.

When you have the majority of your weight on your front leg, a strong sweep or yank will take your whole structure down, whereas, you can buy some time if you had your weight resting on your rear leg instead.

The Wing Chun founders had carefully and cleverly selected the Yijikim Yeungma horse for their fighting system. They designed Siu Nim Tao to help you understand the properties of this horse, and to prepare you to ride it. When you have mastered this form, you are then promoted to the level of a cavalier and taught to ride it and use it as a warhorse. You will learn to depend and fight on it. If you don't understand your horse, you will fall and fail. You must learn to become one with your horse. You can only be as good a cavalier as the horse you ride; and the horse can only ever be as good as its rider.

ELEVEN

FORCE: THE SCIENCE OF PHYSICS AND THE ESSENCE OF WING CHUN

A NIMALS SURVIVE BY THE use of their instincts, which are hard-wired into them at birth. Human beings aren't so fortunate; we have few, if any instincts, and must acquire our knowledge gradually. Most animals can survive well on their own one year after birth; a human child can't survive on his own until he is a teenager. An animal has built-in weapons; tigers have teeth and claws, elephants have brute power and tremendous size, and gorillas are possessed of tremendous strength. Our greatest strength and, indeed, our greatest weapon, is human intellect.

The mind lifted us out of the jungles and taught us how to build homes, how to heat them, how to transport water for drinking and sanitation. We have developed concepts and discovered natural laws, such as those manifested in physics, which in turn have improved our ability to survive.

It is really important to understand the laws of physics when learning martial arts, and for the practical purposes of understanding Wing Chun. The laws of physics have always existed, and will always continue to exist. Our ability to better understand and interpret these laws changes, and perhaps the laws also change in time. However, with each important discovery, scientists in future generations will discover more. If scientists had continued to believe that the world was flat, we couldn't have come as far as we have. The more we understand the universal laws, the more we are able use them to our advantage.

For example, with the information that the Wright Brothers had at the time they were able to make the first airplane fly. The laws of physics had always been there, yet no one knew enough to make manned flight a reality. Even during the time of the Wright Brothers there were others who were working on the concept of flight, but it took the Wright brothers to realize it. They were able to make their planes fly because they knew better than others how force worked. Without the knowledge already bestowed upon them by Newton, his peers, and those before and after him on the properties of force, they couldn't have done it. Today, with more understanding of force, we are able to fly heavier planes, rockets, and missiles at faster speeds than they could ever have fathomed.

Similarly, the more we understand about the laws of physics, biomechanics, and human anatomy, the more we will know about the nature of force production and how to apply it, and thus learn how to become better martial artists. By definition, biomechanics is the physical laws of force and motion applied to the human body.

The Wing Chun training program was not designed to fill a practitioner's mind with images of fighting scenarios that he would then need to try and apply in a real-fighting situation. That's wishful thinking, not serious thinking. No fighting techniques could ever cover the infinite possibilities and variables of how a fight can play out. You never know, for example, where and when you will fight because you can never predict in advance how or when you will be attacked. Further, you never know what kind of opponent you might end up fighting with, in what environment, with what kind of weapon, and under what circumstances. Trying to practice a response for a particular situation that you don't even know will take place will not solve the problem. You can't solve problems by carrying a mindful of possible techniques that might be useable. You may take two hundred techniques with you, but not have the one you need for the situation. You need more than that—and that is what Wing Chun trains you for.

Wing Chun trains you in the science of fighting. When you understand the science, then problem solving becomes easy. If you know the technology of auto mechanics, then you will be able to fix a car stranded in the desert by jerry rigging something out of the materials that are available on site. By contrast, if you had learned to fix specific problems using specific tools without studying what underpins auto mechanics, then you wouldn't be able to troubleshoot anything other than what you had done repeatedly in the workshop using computerized tools. Similarly, without learning the science of fighting, which involves human movement, the earth and the laws that govern both, you will never be able to solve unfamiliar problems once they present themselves.

In Wing Chun, it is more important to store bits of information rather than bytes of information. Bits of information are details for each movement such as Tansau (攤手－Extending Arm), Bongsau (膀手－Wing Arm), or Fooksau (伏手－Prostrating Arm). There is a wealth of detailed information on the use of these "tools" that Wing Chun practitioners generally ignore or, at the very least, are not aware of. By not understanding and mastering these tools, the practitioners are unable to apply them singularly or in conjunction with their other tools. Many Wing Chun schools provide bytes of information for students to store in their minds to use against bytes of presupposed situations. Although this type of training has proven not to work, many teachers continue to teach the art this way.

A more effective way of training the student is to provide him with bits of information that he can then work on perfecting. Once he has mastery over each bit of information, he should be able to assemble a bunch together on the fly to fit each unique situation as it presents itself. As long as he hasn't been given corrupt bytes, his natural survival instinct will put the bits together to suit the situation. That also comes about from reading the situation correctly, which is done from making contact with one's opponent—which, as we've seen, is developed from Chisau exercise.

Wing Chun training is different from martial arts that place a heavy emphasis on speed and physical strength. Although these attributes are necessary, they are not the *only* components required for fighting. In Western sports, such as those in the Olympics, the athletes compete mostly in speed and strength events. In Chinese martial arts, a high-caliber practitioner is not complimented for his speed or physical strength, but for his skills and inner strength. A Chinese person would never say, "Wow! He's fast," or "Wow! He's so (muscularly) strong!" Instead, he'd say, "Wow! He's developed excellent skills," or "Wow! He's got amazing inner strength." In fact, the very word "kung fu" (功夫) is a misnomer that has been applied to all Chinese martial arts. Martial arts were traditionally referred to as wugong (武功), or wushu (武术); civilian fighting arts were referred to as quanfa (*chuenfa*－拳法), meaning, "way (methodology) of the fists (usage)." Kung fu just means skill in the context of achievement through laborious, dedicated, and diligent training. So, when one is said to have "good kung fu," or "good neigong" (內功 inner strength), he is being complimented for the time and effort he has spent in his training in order to have achieved his goals. Speed and physical strength are of lesser importance because of their impermanence; i.e., they are just as easy to lose as to acquire. As they typically decline with age, their shelf life is short in the grand scheme of things, whereas skills that were acquired through years and decades of hard dedicated work will not only last a lifetime, but will actually get better with time.

And this is why Wing Chun is not a "fighting style." For that matter, not one of the martial arts is a fighting style either. Those who enter their martial arts training with the belief that they will soon be shown some special combinational and scenario-based fighting techniques that will allow them to successfully handle similar situations soon find out that they're unable to apply these techniques anywhere, anytime, and with anyone outside of those they attend class with at their martial arts school. At best, they will have learned some bits of information such as basic blocking, punching and kicking that they will be able to use effectively and instinctively in real fighting situations. All the fancy choreographed scenario-based practices will most likely prove ineffective.

THE MISDIRECTED RISE OF MMA

Many martial artists received such a rude awakening after the martial arts boom of the late seventies and early eighties when people were starting to see that not all martial artists could successfully handle aggressive street fighters or grapplers. As a result, they looked in the wrong place for the answer to this problem—instead of looking at the concept underpinning all successful human fighting (i.e., natural laws and physics), they simply adopted more techniques from the grappling arts and thus began the Mixed Martial Arts (MMA) approach. MMA schools then began popping up everywhere, particularly with the promotion this approach received through the widely-distributed Ultimate Fighting Championship (UFC). However, the practitioners of MMA will still have the same problem as long as they treat what they are doing as a style.

Again, there can be no fighting styles because fighting itself has no particular shape or form. One fight will never be like another. It will never be anything like a sparring session in the dojo or a choreographed fight scene in the movies. The environment, circumstances, opponent's height, weight, strength and skills will determine how the fight will look and end. There are far too many variables to ever be able to condense what happens in a real fight into a style.

So, if Wing Chun and other martial arts are not fighting styles, then what are they? They are, one and all, simply training programs for preparing the practitioner to overcome an opponent in a fight based upon the concepts of what a real fight entails according to the founders of each of the arts. Each concept and training method will differ and yet have a commonality. Some concepts will be richer than others. Some training methods will be more practical than others. However, the best system will not necessarily produce the best fighters. Much will depend on the trainer and the trainee. For instance, each automobile manufacturer competes to make the best car in a certain category. For fast cars, there is the Ferrari, Maserati, Porsche, or Lotus. The manufacturers know better than to just make a car that drives fast for that particular consumer market; they have to make it aesthetically beautiful, durable, comfortable, and economical (the best bang for the buck). In other words, it must be holistic. By the same token, there exist other car manufacturers attempting to capture the same market, but they are unable to come up with a product that is as holistic or complete. The difference is in the personnel involved in creating the concept, developing the design, engineering the mechanics, and building it to exacting specifications. Without such personnel, the product will never reach such perfection. However, even with such perfection, not everyone will be able to maintain or raise the quality of the car to its maximum potential. It takes a special person to keep that car looking and running as good as it did when it first came out from the production line. It also takes a special person to be able to drive it at top speeds or win a race with it. These special people may have been born with some inherent talents, but overall, they had to acquire their skills through training, whether from personal experience or from good teachers. To maintain and run the car most effectively, the person operating it must know the car as well as its designers and engineers do. Only then can his talent play a role in bringing out the full potential of the car.

Similarly, different individuals created different martial arts for different purposes. However, some were more ingenious than others. Great martial arts concepts were created over the centuries, however without the right coach and student, none of these arts can be fully realized to their maximum potential. The student must have the mental, physical, and emotional strength to train properly in order to become a top martial artist.

So, what makes a car run more powerfully (pound-for-pound) than another car? What makes a martial artist more powerful (pound-for-pound) than another martial artist?

For the car, it is the designers' and engineers' supreme knowledge of auto mechanics and force. For the martial artist, it is his supreme knowledge of biomechanics and force.

THE PROPERTIES OF FORCE

Let's now look at the properties of Force.

Force, in Physics, is any influence that accelerates an object. An object can experience a force because of the influence of a field, such as with electricity, magnetism, or gravity. Force can be expressed as a vector, meaning that it has both direction and measurable amount. When several forces act on an object, the forces are combined. The total force acting on an object, the object's mass, and the acceleration of the object are all related to each other by Newton's second law of motion. This law states that the total force acting on an object is equal to that object's acceleration multiplied by its mass. Thus, if an identical force acts on two objects of different mass, the one with a larger mass will have a lower acceleration.

Energy, in Physics, is the property of matter that has the capacity to perform work such as motion or the interaction of molecules.

Kinesiology is the scientific study of human movement in terms of physiological, mechanical, and psychological mechanisms. In other words, it is the study of the workings of energy and force in human beings, or the study of biomechanics. It is a relatively new branch of human science that is still being explored, which is somewhat different from how rigid-body mechanisms work when tensegrity is taken into consideration. For this reason, to this day, no one has been able to create a robot that can walk and run freely like a human.

MORE ON POTENTIAL AND KINETIC ENERGY

We take our walking and running abilities for granted, and don't give it a second thought. However, there are kinesiologists who are still trying to figure out the full mechanism of walking. Giovanni Cavagna is a physiologist from the University of Milan; he has been trying to understand the physics of walking for the past forty-five years. He figured that we walk like a pendulum to save energy; however, we do it badly.

In the July 2001 issue of *Discovery Magazine*, in the article titled "The Physics of...Walking," Robert Kunzig writes that Giovanni Cavagna learned that most humans walk inefficiently, delivering about sixty-five percent of what a perfect pendulum could produce; losing thirty-five percent of energy with each step because of the lack of coordination. Much energy is wasted fueling muscular contraction, cooling the body, rubbing muscle fibers and pulling them apart. In some experiments that he and his colleagues did with Kenyan women, he was able to figure out at which point of the stride energy is lost the most. The women were able to walk and carry on their heads seventy percent of their body weight, whereas, his colleagues weren't able to carry more than fifteen percent of their body weight. Surprisingly, the women were able to carry twenty percent of their weight without using any more oxygen or burning any more calories than when they carried nothing. The researchers used a platform that could record the forces exerted by the feet, and measure the potential and kinetic energy at each point of a person's stride. The women did far better than the researchers. Cavagna's team found that the team members on the platform paused momentarily for a few milliseconds as they moved from the top of one stride onto the next. What happens at that moment is that potential energy is lost and not converted to increased speed because the leg muscles contract and resist the fall. Without carrying any load, the women paused between strides; however, when they carried a heavy load on their heads, they were able to shorten or even eliminate the pause, thus, converting more potential energy into kinetic motion, instead of muscle heat. The conversion rate of their gait rose between sixty-five to eighty percent—making them better pendulums than the researchers.

It is important to understand how potential energy converts to kinetic energy and back, and how efficient things can be if the conversion rate was 100 percent. Because of the lack of coordination and resistance caused by opposing muscle groups, humans generally walk inefficiently. Therefore, if we can figure out a way of using only the muscles required to get a job done, and not letting opposing muscles interfere with them, and to fire the different working muscles in the proper sequence (thus accomplishing optimal coordination) to allow full conversion of potential and kinetic energy, then we should be able to deliver an efficient and powerful force. And this is especially true when delivering a punch with optimum explosiveness.

DEVELOPING AN EXPLOSIVE PUNCH

Perhaps the biggest myth about developing a powerful punch is the belief that one must "explode" the punch into the target or point of contact at the very last second. Mark my words as being the first one to say this: The power of a punch is generated at the *beginning* of the punch and not at the end. A projectile such as a bullet, an arrow, or a catapult gains momentum as it begins to propel forward. When it hits a hard surface there will be an *impact*—but not an *explosion*. The harder the surface it hits, the bigger the impact. The softer the surface it hits, the smaller the impact. If the projectile hits nothing, it will neither have an impact nor an explosion. Our bodies can't explode. The closest thing that we can do to simulate this phenomenon is to contract our muscles suddenly and relax them immediately, or suddenly convert potential energy into kinetic energy.

When we decide to punch, certain muscles contract to move our bones towards the target. Our training will determine which muscles will be activated and in what sequence to achieve the desired result. If you've been training to "explode" your punch at the end of your strike, then you will contract your muscles at the end—but which muscles?

In order to propel the arm, you would have already contracted muscles that are necessary to extend the arm. To achieve the objective of extending the forearm towards the target you would need to have contracted your triceps muscle on the back of the upper arm, as that is their function. The biceps (on the front of the upper arm) would have had to relax to let the arm extend. If activated, being responsible for bending the arm toward the body, they would act counter to the function of the triceps muscles and put the brakes on the process of extending the forearm (if contracted equally as forcefully as the triceps) or reduce the strength and speed of the forearm traveling toward your opponent (if contracted with slightly less force than the triceps). So, in order to extend the forearm toward the target with as much strength and speed as possible, you would need to be able to quickly contract your triceps muscle to 100 percent of its capacity and disengage the biceps 100 percent. Another way of explaining this action is that you would activate and deplete your stored potential energy suddenly, by converting it to kinetic energy.

Potential energy is measured by both its position and its mass; whereas kinetic energy is measured by its velocity and mass. When the potential energy is 100 percent, the kinetic is at 0. Conversely, when kinetic energy is at 100 percent, the potential energy is at 0, provided there are no dissipative or counter forces at work. When a body collides with another body, it will transfer its energy to it. The amount of force exerted by the first body onto the second body will be rebounded equally in the opposite direction. That is called impact.

So, if the triceps and other muscles involved in throwing a punch (i.e., the deltoids, pectorals, etc.) were already activated a hundred percent, what would be left to contract? Only the antagonistic muscles to ones necessary for delivering a punch. How would that help? Remember, the bones are what make the contact. By tightening up as many muscles as possible you will only make the muscles harder; doing so won't make the strike any harder. In fact, what these practitioners conceive as an explosion is actually an implosion. Instead of releasing the force, more often than not they're simply pulling it back.

Apart from misconstruing the contraction of flexing muscles as contributing to making one's punch more explosive, if you have in mind to only have this "explosion" take place at the very end, then you are predetermining a specific distance that is required for your hand to traverse prior to the explosion taking place. For example, if you determine to create this explosion at arm's length (i.e., approximately 24 inches from the starting point of the punch), what will you do when if opponent moves in closer to you by 10 inches or moves one-inch back? Your explosion will not take place because your pre-calculation no longer fits the situation, throwing off both the end distance of the punch and its timing. However, if you've already exploded your punch in the beginning, any object that it hits within your arm's length will receive maximum impact.

COORDINATED AND COMBINED FORCE

The posture you assume, the muscles you use, and in what sequence you use them, will determine how much power you will deliver in your punch. Proper sequence will build accumulative force just like multiple levers or gears. Poor posture and incorrect muscle usage will reduce the power of your strikes. Although your subconscious mind knows what muscles to fire sequentially and will do so, your conscious mind will often interfere and fire the inappropriate ones or diminish the involvement of the correct ones because of improper training and mindset.

To generate force from the ground, your structure must be upright and your upper-torso weight placed predominantly onto your rear leg. The more weight you have on the leg supporting the punch, the more weight you will have behind the punch, and the more impact you can create.

To draw force from the ground, you must first contract the abdominal and frontal pelvic muscles, followed by the frontal thigh and calf muscles. This sequence of contraction will extend your leg towards the ground. The generated force will bounce up and raise the structure of your frame vertically (if you have your leg's rear flexing muscles, or hamstrings, relaxed). However, if you engage your leg's rear flexing muscles right after you have contracted the muscles on your frontal thighs, and sequentially move up from your calves to your buttocks, you will restrict the leg from extending and prevent it from raising the structure upward. Instead, you must direct the bounced force from the ground and add onto the force generated by the rear pelvic and back muscles (for rotating the structure) to propel the arm and fist forward.

The fist and forearm should be used only as a projectile batted into motion by the upper arm, which is powered by the grounded structure. If the upper arm flexors (biceps) are activated too strongly in the attempt to generate power, such as by tightening the arm or quickly drawing the arm back a brief distance toward the body at the very end of the punch to create a "snapping" (conceived as explosion by some practitioners) effect, the propelling and kinetic force will be terminated prematurely.

When the fist lands on a target, there will be an impact; the density of the target will determine the amount of impact (returned force). How thorough an impact will be created by the one strike will be determined by how stable you and your opponent are. If your punch drove your opponent five steps back, or drove you back one step, there would, in essence, be just surface impact. However, if you ground your structure solidly, and punched in a way that didn't drive him back five steps, there will be much more thorough and penetrating impact.

Let me provide you with an analogy. If you place a golf ball on a tee and strike it with a hammer in the same fashion that you would with a golf club, the golf ball will fly into the air undamaged. But now, tape that same golf ball to the tee and place the tee in the ground, and then hammer it straight down with your hammer. Smasho! What happens here is that the hammer's force travels through the golf ball and hits the ground, and then bounces back to the hammer, and returns back to the ground—back and forth multiple times in millionth of a second—causing considerable damage to the golf ball. So, don't be overly impressed with a punch that drives a person five steps back. With all the fights I've seen live or on TV, I've never seen anyone stumble back five steps and then fall down as a result of being knocked out cold. Have you? Knockouts are always achieved on the spot or driving the opponent back one step at most.

Wing Chun practitioners talk about their sun (vertical fist) punch as if it is something very unique and deadly but aren't able to do anything with it when put to test. They talk about jerking the fist upward at the end of the hit, exploding the punch at contact, or using the pinky knuckle for striking, but have been routinely put on their butts when they attempt this against boxers. They talk about punching straight (being the shortest path from A to B) but then hammer the fist in a semi-circular motion downward, or swing back their fists horizontally, or swing their whole arm in a semi-circle upward.

In reality, the Wing Chun punch is not that dissimilar from a boxer's punch. It shares the commonality of exploding the punch at the beginning and utilizing kinetic force fully. Although most boxers are trained to rotate their fists and strike when the fist is horizontal these days, they subconsciously punch with their fists at a 45-degree angle (thumb rotated inward). In the early days of boxing, boxers such as Jack Dempsey punched with their fists in a vertical position. Considering the young age of the sport of boxing, I believe Asian martial arts may have influenced boxers to use a horizontal fist position when punching. I believe that boxers punch with 45-degree angled fist because the intuitive (right) brain wants to go vertical, but the analytic (left) brain tells them to go horizontal. So in the ring, the brains meet halfway, and rotates the fist halfway.

The main difference between boxing and Wing Chun punching is the posture. Because boxing rules disallow grappling, kicking, and takedowns, boxers can lean forward when punching with impunity. This gives them body kinetic force behind their punches. Whereas, Wing Chun is a combative art rather than a sport, and so must be able to defend against grappling, kicking, and takedowns. As a result, an upright structure becomes more logical and practical. This doesn't mean that Wing Chun doesn't use body kinetic force; it just employs it differently than boxers do. Instead of rotating with a lean, Wing Chun practitioners rotate while in an upright position. This allows the Wing Chun practitioner to draw more force from the ground through the rear supportive leg. When you lean forward onto the front leg, and lift the heel off the rear foot, some of the kinetic force is brought to the front leg instead of delivering it all to the fist, as there will be less connection from the ground to the fist and vice versa.

Grounding is of utmost importance to a martial artist. The ground assists by generating force against an opponent. When a punch is executed correctly, it will not only travel straight, but also deliver a downward force to the ground to a very deep impact.

The shortest distance from one vertical plane to another vertical plane is a straight line drawn from one point of the vertical plane to the other vertical plane on *one horizontal plane* (not another horizontal plane; otherwise it will travel on an incline or decline, which would be longer in distance). So, a punch traveling upward or downward is not shorter, faster or more direct than a hook punch, which some Wing Chun practitioners like to claim.

To execute the shortest, fastest and most direct hit, the punch must start and end in the same horizontal plane. So, if you want to hit the face, then your fist should be placed at your opponent's face height. Or if your fist is at the solar plexus height, you will generate more impact if you punch your opponent's solar plexus instead of his face. This is not to say that every punch must be done this way, but that this principle will provide you with the most direct, strongest and fastest strike. Additionally, if the correct muscles, sequence, posture, and rotation are used with this alignment, you will deliver even more power. Using the structural alignment proposed by Wing Chun training, you will be able to draw power from the ground and create a very penetrating impact.

Look at the mechanics of the arm for a vertical punch hitting a target beginning and ending on the same horizontal plane. The upper arm is designed to swing in different directions from the shoulder socket. To propel it forward, it swings upward. If you fix the elbow in a bent position, the upper arm will push the forearm and fist upward. In order to make the fist travel in the same horizontal plane, you need to open the elbow and lower the forearm and fist to compensate for the upward-moving force of the upper arm. So, in essence, the fist will be traveling and hitting downwards.

It is essential to time and control the fist drop; otherwise it becomes a hammer swing instead of a thrust.

With the controlled downward hit, the force is sent downward through the opponent's body to his heels and ground, and bounced back up to your fist. If you had punched with the correct posture, muscles and sequence, and if you kept your shoulders relaxed, you would be able to direct the force down to the heel of your supporting leg and bounce the force back from the ground to the fist and through the opponent to his heels again, and, thus, create multiple impacts. *That* would likely create the knockout punch.

However, if you tense your arm and shoulder at the end of the hit, the bounced force from the opponent would pass through your arm and shoulder, and likely jolt you back, thus not allowing you to generate multiple impacts. Also, if you did not release your force kinetically at full capacity, the punch would have the effect of a push, and just stagger the opponent back, not allowing the force to go down to the ground and create the multiple impacts.

The human body has stored energy that we call potential energy. We can use it in three ways. We can supply the energy to our muscles to move our bones to either push or pull (extend or flex) in one form or another. In either case, they deliver force. If there is no external resistance acting upon the force (other than friction), the potential energy can be converted to nearly full kinetic energy; the rate of conversion will depend on how well each individual can transfer potential to kinetic by minimizing the resistance from antagonistic muscles for each required action. This is one of the factors that makes a person a stronger and faster runner, swimmer, or puncher than another person. A human being has 230 movable and semi-movable joints. Whether you are running, swinging a golf club, or punching, you will require the use of your muscles, bones, and joints to accomplish the job. Your potential energy will need to fuel each group of muscles to move the different bones. So if you fuel the contraction of muscles that are not necessary to accomplish your objective, you will not only waste your energy, but will make those muscles work against the ones that are doing the real job. If the potential energy is not allowed to be delivered completely to one set of muscles then it will not provide enough energy to convert itself to 100 percent kinetic energy; subsequently, it will not have the 100 percent kinetic energy to convert to 100 percent potential energy for the next set of muscles that you will need to engage. Consequently, by the time the conversion reaches the last set of muscles you require, it will no longer be powerful. Therefore, the economical and efficient use of energy is vital in delivering force.

While the power of kinetic energy can be felt upon the direct impact of the projectile hitting another object (such as a foot pounding the ground in the case of a runner, a golf ball striking a tree, or a fist hitting a jaw) it is vulnerable to sideswipes, which is why during flight or when in a state of momentum, a plane might wobble in turbulence or a runner might tumble from a slight trip, a golf ball might hook or slice from a deviation in the club swing, and a punch can be deflected by a slight slap. It is important to know this. You must not direct your force directly against a kinetically traveling projectile such as an overhead arm strike, or defend against a pole strike with a rising forearm block. The larger mass will in such a scenario always overpower the lesser one. You can see several examples of how the shin snaps easily against the knee in UFC fights. When you understand the vulnerability of kinetically traveling force during flight, you can then redirect such a force with very little effort. In Wing Chun, it this is called "soft force."

SOFT FORCE

For the Qi-based martial arts such as Tai Chi, Bagua, and Xinyi, Qi (*chee* 氣—air) is referred to as soft force, and muscle-generated force is referred to as hard force. Wing Chun also delves into Qi, but it does not focus on it as heavily as these arts. I believe the Wing Chun founders realized how difficult it was for someone to discover the Qi within oneself and apply it. In the history of martial arts, there have been very few masters who've really reached that level of mastery where they were able to minimize physical strength and maximize Qi power. There may have been a few others who may have reached an infancy stage of this skill, but many who've claimed mastery over it were fakes. Even today, we have these fakes performing their bogus acts under the label of Qigong (*Chi Kung*—氣功).

I believe that the Wing Chun founders took that into consideration when designing the system. They were realists who figured that if someone spent enough time training in martial arts they would learn to manage their energy better, and perhaps one day learn to master Qigong. However, in the meantime, the system needed both a realistic and scientific method of dealing with physical force. Therefore, instead of only considering Qigong as a soft force, the Wing Chun founders decided that any force that neutralizes, deflects or dissolves another force can also be called soft force.

How do you neutralize, deflect, or dissolve a force? Remember that a force is an effort that causes change to an object in its movement, direction, or shape (if flexible). A force, possessing magnitude and direction, is measurable as mass multiplied by acceleration (Newton's formula: F=ma). If the object's mass is constant, its velocity is proportional to the net force acting on it, and inversely proportional to its mass. In other words, the more force you apply to an object, the faster it will accelerate; however, if one object has a larger mass than another, it will accelerate less than the smaller mass when the same amount of force is applied. A thrust in the same direction of the moving object increases the velocity; whereas, a force moving against the traveling object will create drag and decrease its velocity.

When all forces acting upon an object are balanced, the object is in a state of equilibrium. For example, if the leftward force on the object is equal to the rightward force, and the upward force is equal to the downward force (not necessarily having the horizontal force equal to the vertical force), then the object can be said to be at equilibrium. Therefore, if the object is at equilibrium, then the forces are balanced; i.e., the net force is "zero," and the acceleration is zero m/s^2 (meters per second squared). It is also important to note that an object at equilibrium is not necessarily at rest (static equilibrium); it can be in motion and continue in motion at the same speed and direction. Force is measured in Newton units (magnitude) plus a reference to direction; for example, you'd say that the force was 10.0N downward. (One Newton is the amount of force required to cause one-kilogram of mass to accelerate 1m/s^2.)

Although you will need to know the exact amount of force that will be brought to bear on a structure when constructing a building or bridge, you obviously will not be able to mathematically measure your opponent's force against yours. However, it can be measured to a large degree by "feeling." This is where your Chisau training comes into play. One of the main purposes of Chisau training is to teach the student how to read and measure force from feeling. We have a general sense for it when dealing with static objects but not so good with moving objects. For example, we're able to visually judge and put out just the right amount of force to pick up a dumbbell off the floor or pull open a door, but we require some training in order to catch a baseball without hurting our hand. The problem with depending solely on our visual sense is that it can be deceived quite easily. Magicians do this to us all the time. In daily life, we often misjudge the weight of an unfamiliar door and push it or pull it too hard. If a fake dumbbell weighing 250 grams was labeled 5 kilograms, and you lifted it thinking it so, you'd probably look pretty silly flying back with your arm swinging overhead and landing on your butt.

The best way to prevent such a misjudgment is to add tactile sense to the reading. If you grabbed the handle of the door or the dumbbell first with the intent of measuring the resistance from 0.0N (equilibrium state) and then increasing the force incrementally and minutely, you would then not be as likely to make the same miscalculation you would have with simply a visual reading and applying a miscalculated force. Blind people probably never misjudge the weight of a door or a dumbbell because they are not deceived by their visual judgment and preconceptions. In essence, they always calculate the weight tactilely first before applying the measured force.

When catching a fast flying baseball, you will also need the tactile sense in addition to the visual one in order to stop it without hurting your hand. You need to neutralize the incoming force by moving your hand, at the point of contact, at the same speed and direction as the traveling ball first before slowing it down and changing direction. In Wing Chun, you should deal with an incoming force similarly instead of stopping it directly with impact. Let's look at how we can neutralize, deflect, and dissolve an incoming force, and what the differences are between these three.

BLOCKING FORCE

Let's say for example that your opponent's arm weighs 2 kg, and he exerts a 2 N force to deliver a punch at 1 m/s^2 traveling from north towards south. Let's also say that your arm weighs 1 kg, or half the weight of his arm. You will need just half the amount of force to deliver the same velocity, i.e. 1-N force to accelerate 1-kg mass at 1 m/s^2. If you were to catch his punch directly with your hand traveling from south to north, his punch will drive your hand back and would probably result in your hitting your own your face with the back of your own hand because his arm has more mass than yours. If you applied more Newton force than his, thus delivering more velocity than 1 m/s^2, the impact may stop the punch but you'd likely hurt your hand because his arm's mass is bigger. Therefore, dealing with an incoming force directly is not wise. Boxers often block punches directly; however, both competitors wear heavily padded gloves so they don't hurt their hands when they're hit, or hurt their faces when the opponent's punches pushes their own gloves to their faces.

Another blocking technique commonly taught in martial arts is to drive the forearm upwards directly against an incoming overhead or horizontal strike such as a "Karate Chop" or to block a downwards blow made with a wooden staff. Here again, the smaller mass will suffer. No matter how much you condition your forearms you will feel a lot of pain or break your forearm bones doing this. Those Wing Chun schools that drill their students to bang each other's forearms for the purpose of "hardening them up" will only make their students suffer bruises and arthritic pain in their later years. Those drills are absolutely unnecessary, and are totally against the principles of Wing Chun.

DEFLECTION FORCE

Many martial art styles will block an incoming strike by swinging your arm and striking his arm from a 90-degree angle, i.e., swinging your arm from east to west or west to east, like many martial arts systems do. Although this action will deflect the punch, it is a 100 percent defensive technique; it doesn't embody Wing Chun's principle of always incorporating offense in with defense, or always directing your arm towards the opponent's Centerline, and economizing your action. Whether you block a punch directly or strike it from a 90-degree angle, Wing Chun considers that as unnecessary hard force. Such techniques are not economical, efficient or productive.

NEUTRALIZATION AND DEFLECTION

In Wing Chun there are several better, more economical, and efficient ways of dealing with a straight incoming punch. For instance, you can slice the incoming punch with a Paksau (拍手—Clapping Hand) from a very acute angle and "brake" it just like the rubber pad of a bicycle gripping the wheel's rim. A bicycle's brake is placed just 2 millimeters away from the rim, and is shaped to conform to the rim. Its job is not to put a sudden stop to the spinning wheel, since such an action would throw the rider frontally off the bike; instead, it uses friction to slow down the speed of the spinning wheel quickly. In essence, the brake first connects to the rim to measure the force and increases its force incrementally to match that of the wheel and finally comes to the point of neutrality or equilibrium, which causes the wheel to stop spinning, or come to rest. Similarly, the Paksau hand travels close to the punching arm, making contact, and applying a brake to the force until it comes to rest. It is important to understand that your arm will always travel at an angle even though the hand is directed along the Centerline Plane. This is because your arm protrudes from your shoulders on the sides of your body frame and not from the middle of your chest. So, when you place your Wusau (guarding hands) in your Centerline Plane and let your upper arms hang down in a relaxed manner, your upper arms will be approximately 90 degrees from your coronal plane and your forearms will angle approximately 45 degrees from your coronal plane, and each of your hands will intersect the Centerline Plane at approximately 22.5 degrees, with both hands forming approximately a 45-degree angle. All of these angles are inherently strong in terms of their structure. To further strengthen the arm structure, the upper arm and forearm (elbow) angle should be set more or less at 135 degrees.

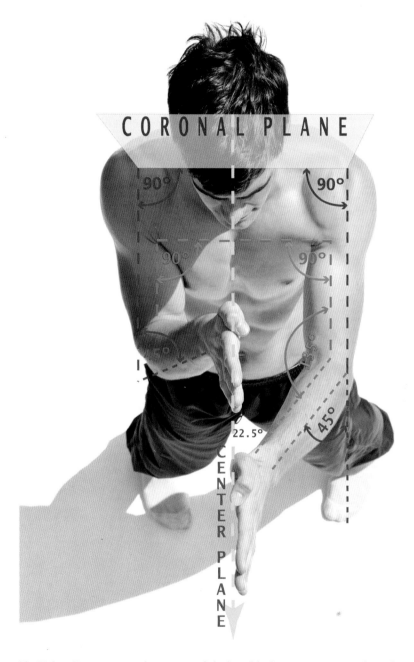

The Yijikim Yeungma en-garde posture with body and limbs in approximate right-angles and 45-degree angles

The hand of the Paksau moves along your Centerline Plane to the opponent's Centerline. All the angles mentioned above change minutely. Because the opponent's punching arm is already in motion, your secondary Paksau force, coming from any angle will easily deflect the punch, provided your arm is not significantly smaller in mass than the opponent's (such as that of a child's against an adult's) or travelling much slower in velocity than that of the opponent's punch. The narrower you angle your force against his incoming force, the lesser you will deflect the punch angularly. The larger you angle your force, the more angular the punch will deflect. Billiard players know that too well. The fact is that you don't need to or want to deliver too much force or deflection. You just need to move the punch out of harm's way. By braking and matching the force of the punch at a small angle, you will deflect his forward-punching force that's aimed at your Centerline, to move it just outside of it. Your Paksau, when directed to your opponent's Centerline will now occupy the Centerline Plane. This is a huge advantage because your hand will now be aimed at his Centerline. Additionally, because of the braking action instead of a striking action, your hand will still be in contact with your opponent's so you can detect any changes on his part, and control them to your advantage. All of this can be done as a result of a small economical and efficient action, which can produce a very advantageous result.

One thing to note is that the literal translation for Paksau (拍手) is "Clapping Hand." The Wing Chun founders chose the words carefully to describe the action specifically. Many practitioners translate Paksau as "Slapping Hand" and do exactly that. However, slapping or swatting is a swinging action, whereas clapping is a light hand beat using a soft wrist action. In fact, when done correctly, it will sound exactly like a clap, not a thud or a slap.

Moreover, it is important to realize when doing Paksau, whether as a drill or in sparring, that you are not intentionally clapping or intercepting the opponent's forearm, wrist or elbow with your inside palm, but that you are intercepting, because both your palm and his punch are traveling towards each other's Centerline. When he attacks your Centerline, your intended response is to probe and/or attack his Centerline with your hand—not to stop his punch. Your hand or forearm just happens to intercept his arm because both of you are traveling along the same path but arriving from different directions. If there is no interception, then it becomes a strike. If there is a small interception, such as your forearm crossing his, you may continue your attack and make the forearm connection work as a defensive check against his attack. If your hand happens to connect to any part of his arm, then it will act as a neutralizer to brake his force. Your Paksau

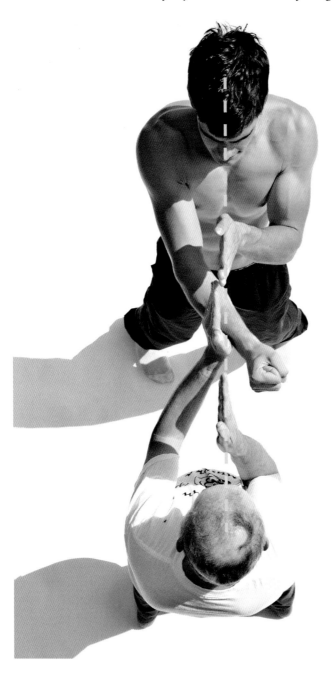

David directs his Paksau toward Isaac's Centerline, thus deflects Isaac's punch from his own Centerline.

will come to a stop just because his arm is in the way of your path. This doesn't mean that you stop exerting any force. Neutrality doesn't mean no force, but that equal forces acting upon each other in opposite directions have canceled each other out to reach a balanced force. Therefore, you must apply via your hand on your opponent's arm the same amount of force that caused the neutrality—no more and no less. If he decreases his force, then you may increase it to neutralize it or direct it elsewhere to create an opening to finish your attack. What you must not do, which is commonly done by many Wing Chun practitioners and other martial artists, is to neutralize your own force by applying biceps and triceps force equally and bringing your arm to a static position.

Paksau, when done correctly, neutralizes the opponent's punch and creates openings for your attack. For that matter, Tansau, Fooksau, Bongsau, and all the other Wing Chun actions can or should be done that way; i.e., used for neutralizing and opening paths for successful attacks.

NEUTRALIZATION AND DIFFUSION

To deflect an incoming force, you don't always have to apply force from the opposite direction; and neither do you need to remain static to stay neutralized. Remember that an object can be in equilibrium and still be in motion. For example, a motorcycle tied to the bed of a moving pickup truck is at rest (equilibrium) as a result of the forces of the straps securing it being tied and pulled in opposite directions. Although it is static, it is also in motion; you can verify that by slamming on the brakes of the truck and observing how the motorcycle will continue its forward motion.

In Wing Chun, we can also neutralize and deflect an incoming force without braking it. It is called "receiving." However, most practitioners don't receive correctly in order to neutralize the force while it's in motion. The training comes from one of the Paksau drills as well as the Chisau exercises. In the Paksau drill, instead of clapping the opponent's arm during travel, you would reach forward with your Wusau to make contact on the outside of your opponent's wrist at the start of the punch in order to calculate his force. As his punch travels towards you, you will match his force (magnitude and direction) with yours by resting your hand on his wrist and following the inward direction until near expiration, at which point you will change the direction. This action will not only take the punch out of harm's way, but will also spread the punch force thin over a longer distance and time. A punch is only good at the point of impact. When it doesn't hit anything, the force is dissipated into nothing. A punching arm can only travel as far as the joints will allow. So, by changing the direction of the punch, its force will diffuse, dissolve, and ultimately expire at the end of his reach. This receiving action can be achieved with all Wing Chun tools such as Tansau, Bongsau, Fooksau, or Gangsau (耕手－Plowing Arm).

The founders of Wing Chun developed the Centerline concept for no other reason than its simple and effective practicality. Most of a human being's vital and vulnerable points are located on the front, back and side centerlines. Therefore, it is logical to strike at your opponent's Centerline and defend your own Centerline. You do this by placing your hands, arms, feet and legs along the Centerline Plane as guards.

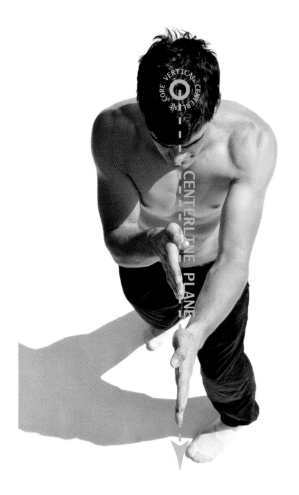

Proper en-garde position will ensure that both hands and feet (rear heel and front toes) touch the Centerline Plane thus protecting one's own Centerline and aiming to attack the opponent's Centerline.

The Centerline Plane is the plane aimed from your Centerline (vertical line drawn from your center core) to your opponent's Centerline. You attack your opponent's Centerline and defend your own Centerline by moving your limbs along the Centerline Plane. By doing so, you are not only attacking the opponent's Centerline along the shortest and most direct path, but also protecting your own Centerline.

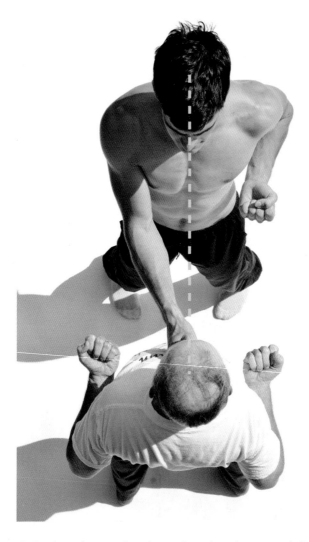

Placing the hands on the Centerline Plane and attacking the opponent's Centerline along the Centerline Plane will render the most direct and shortest line of travel.

With this in mind, you must therefore never direct your opponent's incoming attack sideways, but along the Centerline Plane in an incline or decline. By moving his attack sideways; that is, moving your hand sideways from the Centerline Plane, you will have created an opening for your opponent to attack your Centerline along the Centerline Plane.

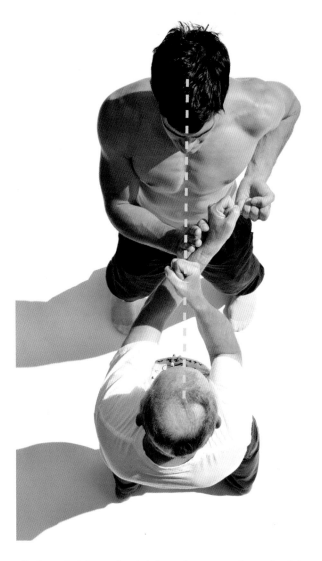

A centrally-directed defensive hand deflects the opponent's punch while remaining in the Centerline Plane—in the way of upcoming attacks.

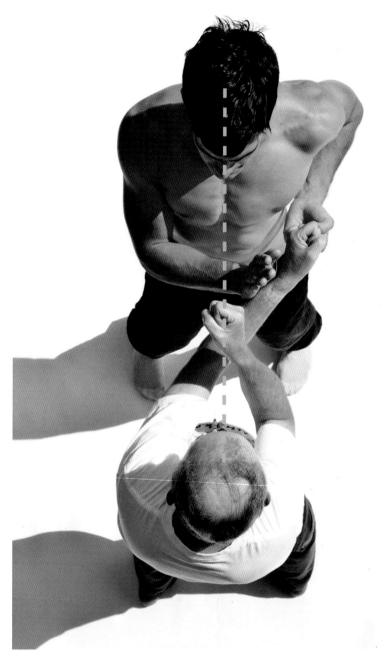

When a defensive hand is directed sideways, it creates an opening for the opponent to direct an attack to the Centerline along the Centerline Plane.

To keep your hand in the Centerline Plane, you can take the opponent's attack upward or downward, which will not only take it out of harm's way, but it will serve to neutralize and diffuse it.

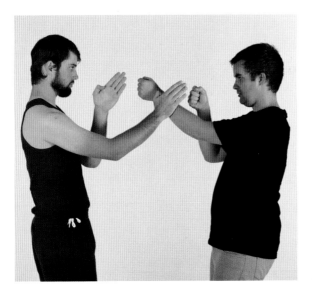

Paksau drill

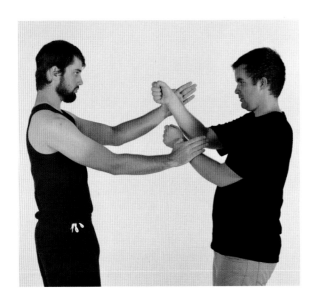

Transform Paksau to Receiving Wusau by reaching out the inside hand towards the partner's punch as it begins travelling.

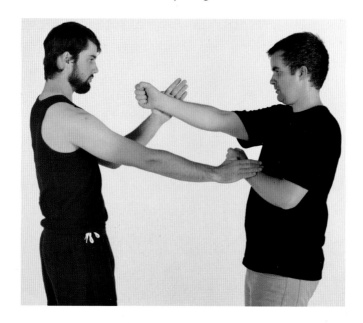

Allow the partner's punch to travel straight—almost to full extension.

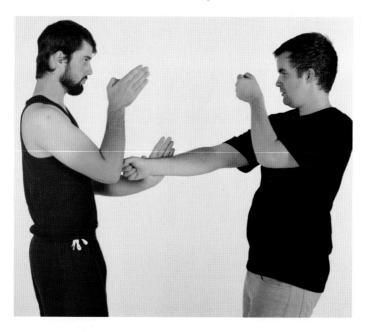

Just before full extension of the punch, drop the Wusau to the solar plexus region; this action takes the punch away from the intended target, out of harm's way, keeps partner's hand in check, and keep own hand on Centerline Plane for defense and/or attack.

For that matter, you could even allow your opponent's strike to come straight through if you've connected to the opponent's arm from the outside. Because the arms originate from the sides, the attacks will always come from an angle to the center; therefore, as long as you receive and bring the contact (your hand on your opponent's arm) to the Centerline Plane, his punch will go to the side of Centerline Plane.

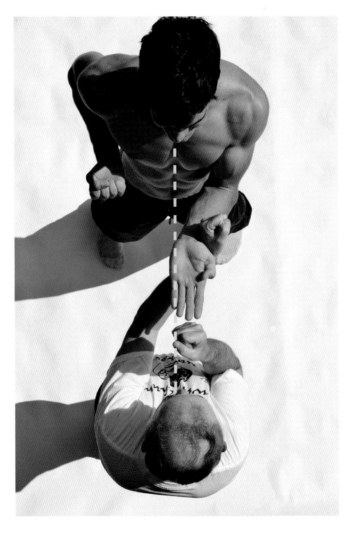

A Receiving Tansau—when stuck to the outside of a punch coming from diagonally across—will take the punch away from the Centerline Plane when the Tansau travels along the Centerline Plane.

Most Wing Chun practitioners treat Paksau drills as repetitive defensive exercises to create muscle memory to deal with incoming punches. The puncher practices his punching, and the defender practices slapping the punch out of the way. Before long, they are doing them mindlessly and mistakenly. The puncher no longer punches straight along the vertical Centerline Plane or horizontal plane. He ends up punching circularly along the vertical plane or swinging outwardly to meet the Paksau. The defender ends up throwing his Paksau before the punch has initiated. He swings his arms across the Centerline Plane and often throws his upper body forward (thus unbalancing himself), and uses his opponent's punching arm as a stabilizer to regain his balance. Practicing this way breaks every Wing Chun principle outlined in the Siu Nim Tau form.

The Paksau drill must be done mindfully. The puncher must shoot each punch individually with a beginning and an end versus continuously in the circular motion. He must initiate the explosion (sudden contraction followed by immediate relaxation) and let the punch fly out freely (kinetically). He must ensure that the punch travels and ends in the same horizontal and vertical planes as its origin. When it is intercepted by any contact, whether it is a Paksau, Tansau, or Bongsau, one must not contract any opposing muscles or resist against the force directly. Instead, one must read one's partner's force and neutralize it. If done correctly, the opponent's strike will be at rest upon the contact.

The Paksau practitioner must also initiate an explosive and kinetic action each time. It must have a beginning and an end (expiration), followed by a resurgent energy (refresh) to begin the next action. The outgoing hand must also travel and end in the same horizontal and vertical planes as the original position. He uses his visual sense to roughly judge how much force is coming towards him and match it with his outgoing force. However, at the point of interception, he must adjust his force to accurately neutralize it.

Let me remind you that the Paksau drill trains you to focus on moving your arms and hands towards your partner's Centerline along the Centerline Plane. You should not focus on slapping or intercepting your partner's incoming punch as a defensive technique. Your objective is to generate an attack with your open-hand Wusau towards your partner's Centerline as soon as you detect an attack coming from your partner. Because your partner is throwing his fist towards your Centerline at your head in the exercise, and you are responding with a counter attack toward his Centerline at his head with your Wusau, they will inevitable intercept. At the point of interception, you will learn to neutralize the forces rather than exert extra force or reduce it. However, in a sparring or real-fighting situation, you may intercept the opponent's punching arm or ride over it with your open-hand or fist to his head, and use your forearm to neutralize his force. There are many ways to deal with an incoming attack; the Paksau exercise merely trains you to respond to an incoming attack with another attack towards the opponent's Centerline, along the Centerline Plane, in a timely manner, and neutralize whatever contact is made in the process.

At this point, you may be saying, "Ah ha, but you said that you shouldn't use your visual sense to judge a force!" No, that is not what I said. I said that the visual sense can be deceiving, and that you must use your tactile sense additionally to measure it correctly. As long as you have the visual sense, you must use it in conjunction with the tactile sense. You do not replace the visual sense with your tactile sense. A blind man may not misjudge the weight of a door or dumbbell, but he certainly will misjudge the direction and force of a baseball coming at him. So, Paksau is not just a mindless slapping drill, but an exercise to train its practitioners on the skills of measuring and neutralizing force. It trains them to execute an action powerfully and accurately. It trains them to convert potential energy to kinetic energy efficiently. Additionally, it trains them to maintain a firm structure, balance, and rooting, which they've learned in Siu Nim Tau, but in this case, applying them while delivering explosive force against another person.

A sifu may begin teaching the Paksau drill right from the start, or after the student completes Section One of the Siu Nim Tau form, or after the student completes all of the Siu Nim Tau form. I don't think the ancient teachers taught the Paksau drill until after the student had completed the Siu Nim Tau successfully; that is, after the student had acquired a solid understanding of it, and had acquired the physical ability to perform it near perfection. Moreover, he may have had to complete the Dan Chisau (打黐手—Single Sticking Arm) exercise successfully as well before moving on to Paksau.

DAN CHISAU EXERCISE

Obviously the ability to neutralize an opponent's force is a big part of Wing Chun's training. It actually begins with Dan Chisau (打黐手—Single Sticking Arm), and progresses to Seung Chisau (雙黐手—Double Sticking Arms) to Chigerk (黐脚—Sticking Leg), onto *all* phases of training. I've accented the word "all" because it is something most Wing Chun practitioners fail to do and even debunk the concept of Chisau in sparring and practical fighting.

Dan Chisau is the fundamental exercise for the sticking concept. If it is not taught or learned properly at this stage, a student will never reach the level of proficiency that the Wing Chun program was designed to do. To many practitioners, the Dan Chisau drill is taught briefly and incorrectly, and then forgotten about. It is considered insignificant and boring for the teachers and students. In reality, it is a very important phase of Wing Chun training. It is the first training exercise, after learning the standalone Siu Nim Tau form, where a student actually makes contact with another student. Remember, the Wing Chun system was not only designed for economical, efficient and productive usage, but its training program itself is likewise designed to foster the attributes of economy, efficiency, and productivity. Therefore, there is nothing useless or insignificant in any part of the training program. Every part is equally useful and significant and can serve to make you a better Wing Chun practitioner.

Most practitioners do the Dan Chisau exercise with vigor and speed. For that matter, they perform all of the Wing Chun forms, exercises, Chisau, and sparring vigorously and rapidly. This may be what is expected and required of other martial arts, but certainly not for Wing Chun. Wing Chun's main training goal is to help the student develop sensitivity and awareness of his surroundings, his own actions, and those of his opponent. By doing things hurriedly and vigorously, he will not read his own actions or his opponent's actions well enough to put himself at a more advantageous position than his opponent. He will also not be prepared for the changes that can occur between the start and the finish of his or his opponent's actions. For this reason, it is important to train slowly to develop awareness of every moment and every movement.

Dan Chisau should be exercised slowly to develop an accurate awareness of one's own force against that of an opponent's. In other words, to learn to measure, neutralize and control all of the forces involved in a combative situation. Dan Chisau is actually an extension of the Siu Nim Tau form, as its movements are extracted directly from the form itself, and incorporates aspects of Yijikim Yeungma, Tansau, Fooksau, Bongsau, Huensau (圈 手−Circling Hand), Jadsau (室手−Braking Hand), Jatji Kuen (日字拳−Sun Fist), and the Pianjoeng (偏掌−Slant Palm) strike. It embodies all of the principles of Wing Chun that are presented in the Siu Nim Tau form, such as the concept of Centerline, Yin-Yang, making offense and defense one entity, maintaining a firm structure but applying soft-arm action, rooting the structure deeply into the ground, always projecting a constant forward force towards the opponent's Centerline, delivering force from the waist down and the waist up, and knowing every moment of your own action. Whilst Siu Nim Tau is exercised alone, Dan Chisau is exercised with a partner. Here, a student is first exposed to physical contact and is introduced to a new set of Wing Chun principles such as the importance of knowing the opponent as much as knowing oneself, becoming one with the opponent, as well as measuring and neutralizing the opponent's force before exerting one's own.

Ideally, Dan Chisau should be taught after fully learning and understanding Siu Nim Tau, and performing it to near perfection. However, with today's lifestyle, no one is patient and dedicated enough to practice only Siu Nim Tau for six to twelve months to achieve this goal. Most schools breeze through Siu Nim Tau and Dan Chisau, and then hustle on into techniques and applications right away without the students first establishing a strong foundation. There is just no way anyone can build upon a weak foundation, whether it is a high-rise tower, an education, or excellence in martial art.

Here is how Dan Chisau should be exercised.

You and your partner should stand squared to each other in the Yijikim Yeungma position about arm's-length apart. Once in this position, your body frames should remain absolutely static; they must not twist or waver to the sides; only your arms will move in this exercise. Your structure must be rooted deeply to the ground by stretching your upper torso, as if the crown of your head wants to touch the ceiling, and sinking your lower trunk as if your knees want to touch the ground. You create this upward and downward tension to apply the principles of Tensegrity to enhance your structure, balance, and rooting.

Before you start, clear all thoughts from your mind and refresh it with the understanding that this exercise is not for developing maximum speed or power; it is not for developing muscle memory for situation-based techniques, and, most of all, it is not a competitive ego game to see who can get through with a hit or score more points. It is an exercise to understand the nature of force, and how you can neutralize it. It helps you find your minimum range of force; i.e., what it takes to get a job done with minimum effort, and it teaches you to read your partner's force and action from your tactile sense.

It is essential that the two of you help each other achieve these goals. The exercise is a partnered effort. Although the two of you are individuals, in this exercise you make yourselves one entity, just like the Yin-Yang philosophy and symbol. The two of you will help each other in feeling and achieving neutrality. You will correct each other when one applies more force than is required. Any imbalance in force must be corrected by reducing the force just enough to bring the two forces back to a state of equilibrium.

Think of your arm as if it were a car with rear wheel drive; and think of your upper arm as the rear wheel, your forearm as the chassis (or the shaft that connects the rear wheel axle to the front wheel axle) and your hand as the front wheel that you will steer in different directions. With this in mind, your upper arm will act as the only force that drives the chassis. The forearm (chassis) and hand (front-wheel mechanism) will take no part in the driving force, but only serve to deliver the force that is generated by the upper arm (the rear wheel mechanism). Presume that you are driving a car called Tansau, and your partner is driving one called Fooksau. We will use this analogy to an extent to demonstrate how to apply a rear-driven force and how to neutralize that incoming force. We cannot use the analogy completely since we will need to steer our arms up and down, which a car cannot do. However, we will use the concept of free frontal steering to demonstrate how we can move our hands with minimum effort and cause the opponent's arm to move in another direction and yet maintain the neutrality between your force and his.

You both begin from the Yijikim Yeungma position with each arm folded on the sides as in the Siu Nim Tau reset position. Say that you are facing north, and that you are sharing the Centerline Plane with your partner; i.e. you both have the same Centerline Plane, and that his Centerline (the perpendicular line running from the crown of the head to ground) is your North, and your Centerline is South to him. In this case, your right fist is positioned at SSE in reference to North, and your left fist is positioned SSW. Open your left hand to form the Tansau shape, i.e. flat palm, thumb bent and tucked to the side of your index finger, and all fingers touching each other to form one unit. Your wrist must be relaxed so it has a small bend at the back of the wrist.

Begin driving your Tansau (car) at an incline towards your partner's Centerline (North), aiming your middle finger at his throat's jugular notch. You apply minimal force with your upper arm to drive the forearm forward, using your hand to steer upward, doing exactly as you would in your Siu Nim Tau form. (Note that many schools move the Tansau parallel to the ground in their Siu Nim Tau form; however, I teach it moving at an incline. I will not explain why at this point, but will do so in a later instructional book on the Siu Nim Tau form.) For the sake of simplicity, I will not talk about Newton force or meters per square second, but just use kilometer per hour for reference to force. So, in this case, we'll refer to the amount of energy you apply (the amount of pressure you apply on the gas pedal) to move your Tansau (car) as the amount that will move it at a speed of 5 km/h, which simply represents a baseline reference for the minimum effort and velocity of your Tansau. Your partner will then initiate his right Fooksau in the same manner; i.e., driving the forearm with his upper arm, using his hand to steer upwards along the Centerline Plane towards your jugular notch at the speed of 5 km/h. His right Fooksau will originate from NNW, and head south.

Because both of you are steering your hands towards each other's jugular notch along the Centerline Plane, your arms will inevitably intercept at a point just outside of the Centerline Plane (left of it from your perspective, and right of it from your partner's perspective). For this exercise, you will allow the Fooksau to ride over your Tansau to intersect and intercept at each other's wrist point, whereby your radial bone at the wrist will connect and pressurize against your partner's radial bone. Because both of you are driving at 5 km/h, your forces will come to a state of equilibrium; i.e. neutrality or state of rest. This is like the friction point that you achieve driving a manual-transmission car—applying just the right amount of gas and clutch pressure to stay stationary on an inclined road. At this point, neither of you should step on your gas pedal to accelerate, which is a common reaction, but rather strive to maintain the original force that continues to generate a 5 km/h velocity. A common reaction at this point is for both trainees to turn their respective engines off and stall at 0 km/h. Although both cars are at rest, there is zero force acting upon each other; therefore, there is no forward force coming from either of you. The point of this exercise is for the Wing Chun student to learn to always have a forward force directed to his opponent's Centerline, and to read his opponent's force. In practical usage,

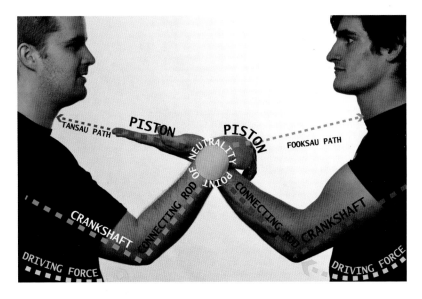

Starting position of Dan Chisau: both participants are in the Yijikim Yeungma posture; Isaac drives left Tansau slowly; Joe drives right Fooksau slowly; both drive to each other's Centerline at an incline towards each other's throats; their wrists intercept and arrive at an equilibrium state because they both drive at the same speed.

when the opponent drops his force, and you feel it, you should then step on the gas to accelerate your Tansau and convert it into a strike. (This will be like releasing the clutch and equally increasing the pressure on the gas from friction point for a manual-transmission car.) The chassis of your car will automatically deflect the opponent's without even intentionally driving the car sideways. However, for the purpose of this exercise, if your partner stops applying force towards your Centerline, you must remind him to accelerate it back to the 5 km/h velocity in order to regain neutrality. On the other hand, if he senses that you've increased your force at this stage, he must tell you to reduce it.

The two of you must hold this feeling of neutrality for some moments to allow your mind to register it. Repeated exercise of this feeling will eventually train your mind to always recognize this state of neutrality. Obviously, you will not always confront your opponent with this amount of force. It will vary, and you will need to adapt to these variations. Also, both of you will not remain static after an interception. The Dan Chisau exercise takes this into account.

So, after the pause, you will initiate a Pian Jeong (偏掌 – Slant Palm) Strike towards your partner's throat. You will now step on the gas and double the speed of your car to 10 km/h. You must push your forearm forward along

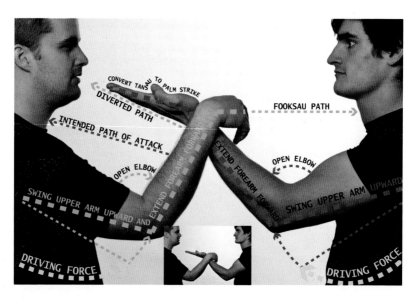

Isaac initiates a supinated palm strike toward Joe's neck; when Joe feels the advancing attack, he extends his Fooksau forward towards Isaac's neck—thus, neutralizing the attack, taking it out of harm's way, and still maintaining his Fooksau on the Centerline Plane.

his point of contact, but create new points of contact along your radial bone in order to move forward. If your partner keeps his force at 5 km/h, his Fooksau will inevitably be pushed aside. Therefore, upon detection of your advancing speed, he must also step on his gas pedal to increase his speed to match yours at 10 km/h. By doing so, he achieves neutrality. Moreover, he maintains neutrality by moving upward with you, maintaining a balanced force but moving it to another position.

What he must *not* do is to try to stop your motion by stopping his own; i.e., by slamming on his brakes (applying both biceps and triceps), or increasing his force to a greater level than yours.

Because you initiated the attack, and he responded secondarily, your contact against his wrist has advanced slightly from your wrist to a point on your forearm just behind the wrist. In the Dan Chisau exercise, it is important to always have one person to initiate an action, and for the other person to react after. This trains you for the reality of a true fighting situation. There is always an action and reaction. Too often, Wing Chun practitioners do this exercise too quickly; consequently, the person who is supposed to react, acts before the person who is supposed to act first. This also happens in the Paksau drills. The Paksau fellow throws his Pak hand before the Puncher throws his punch. In a real fight situation, you

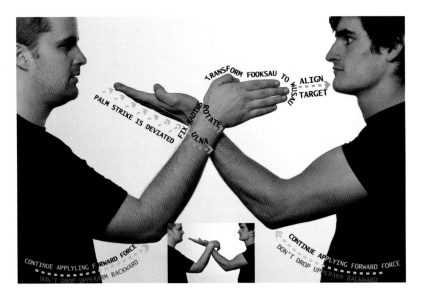

Joe fixes his radius and rotates his ulna underneath to line the palm and fingers along the Centerline Plane towards Isaac's Centerline; in doing so, he lowers Isaac's hand and "routers" it out of the Centerline Plane.

can never be so certain of your opponent's action to predict (and act) upon it. You must always sense it first. This is what Wing Chun trains you for—to read the situation accurately and to respond accurately in a timely manner—in other words, to train your awareness to a very high consciousness level.

In the next part of the drill, your partner will perform exactly what he learned in the Fooksau movement in Siu Nim Tau; i.e. he will drive his Fooksau with his upper arm upward at an incline and, at about chin height, he will rotate his wrist (Huensau) until his baby finger lines up with his ulnar bone, at which point he will pick up each finger to point forward, beginning with his index finger pointing at a spot along the horizontal plane just below his own eyes (about the middle of the length of the nose).

When he has all of his fingers and palm lined up and flush with the Centerline Plane, he will then use his index finger as a fixed point of reference and drop his wrist down vertically (Jadsau).

All through the period of doing the Huensau and Jadsau, the upper arm doesn't stop moving forward. Most Wing Chun practitioners stop the upper arm movement to perform Huensau and Jadsau, but that is akin to turning the engine off or stepping on the brakes and then turning the wheels. The force should be continuous. In the Siu Nim Tau form, it is only when the Jadsau is completed that the upper arm begins to swing back down to retract the Wusau. When done properly, the Fooksau to Huensau to Jadsau to Receiving Wusau and back to Fooksau will convert smoothly (without stopping and starting) and continue without pause. The three-time repetition of the hand-shape conversion is called "The Cycle" for this reason. It's not called "The Stop And Go And Stop And Go And Stop And Go." It's called "The Cycle!"

Now that your partner is performing the above action with physical contact with you, he must make sure to keep his radius and ulna contact pressured against your wrist with the same amount of force that is driving your arms at 10 km/h towards his Centerline at an incline. In effect, he is directing your attack higher than you had intended, out of harm's way. Although he could carry on pushing the contact upward above his head, and, thus, continue to dissipate the force of your attack, he will not gain any particular advantage for the next move by doing so; in fact, he would endanger himself in a real fighting situation by exposing his head to another attack from his opponent's other hand. Therefore, one must know the parameters of how far one can or should drive one's vehicle before it comes dangerous. For this reason, there are markings on roads to show where you can drive and where you cannot. For that matter, most things in life have parameters for good reasons. Similarly, Wing Chun training, whether embedded in the forms or drills will always teach these parameters.

Once the knuckle of your partner's index finger reaches the height of your lips he will begin rotating his wrist (steer his car) to align his fingers to the bridge of your nose, while continuing to push his upper arm forward. In the process of rotating his wrist and lining up his hand vertically to the Centerline, he will fix his radius in one position and rotate the ulna medially (inward), which will push your Tansau out of the Centerline Path. I call the action of fixing one forearm bone and rotating the other to sweep away the opponent's arm as "carving" or "routering," like a carpenter's router tool would do. A carpenter's router blade is shaped like a butterfly with a pointed head. When he starts the motor, the blades spin around the sharp point. He then pushes the point to the axis marking of the door-lock hole he wants to carve out, and the butterfly blade carves out a perfect circle. This is a very effective tool in Wing Chun. In fact, Tansau, Bongsau, Jadsau, Huensau, Gwansau, and Gangsau all have routering properties. Routering action is much more efficient and effective than swinging the forearm sideways from the elbow, or swinging the upper arm sideways from the shoulder joint. These two actions take more energy to perform; moreover, it takes your hand and arm out of the Centerline Plane.

After he aligns his fingers to your Centerline, he fixes his index finger at one spot, and lowers the ulna edge of his wrist to perform Jadsau. He does not raise his fingers up like many Wing Chun practitioners do. He will also not use his triceps to lower his forearm, nor use his latissimus to pull his upper arm back (thus lowering it), or use both in conjunction to lower his whole arm. Instead of using large muscles to create a big action, he only uses the extensors on his forearm to create a small but powerful wrist action to steer your forearm down; just enough to create an opening for his forthcoming attack. Note that his Jadsau should only steer the forearm down rather than be used as a dominant force. It is the upper arm that delivers the dominant force to drive the forearm forward towards your Centerline at 10 km/h.

When you sense his Jadsau pressing down against your Tansau wrist, you must not resist upward, but maintain the neutrality by moving your forearm downward from your elbow while still applying forward pressure from your upper arm that delivers 10 km/h against his 10 km/h. However, you must not lower your upper arm; because by doing so, you will give up the 10 km/h forward force. Remember, it is your upper arm swinging upward that delivers the 10 km/h force. Once you lower it, you are swinging backward, thus, reversing your car or rolling backward on a hill.

Your Tansau arm angle is formed by your biceps pulling up your forearm at an insertion point on the radial bone just in front of the inside elbow joint. When done correctly, it contracts just enough to hold the forearm in position to resist gravity's force. The triceps must be relaxed; otherwise, you will end up contracting your biceps more to resist the triceps' downward pull on your forearm. This is how you will end up with a "tight" arm. Also, your partner must not apply more downward force on your wrist than necessary; otherwise, you will be tempted to contract your biceps more to resist it, and end up with an upward and downward gridlock instead of the even 10 km/h versus 10 km/h forward forces that have come to rest. Therefore, his Jadsau must be light—performed with just his flexors instead of the triceps and/or the latissimus muscles.

In order to maintain this light neutrality, when your partner presses your wrist with his Jadsau, you must release just enough biceps contraction to let your forearm go with his Jadsau in real time (real time in this example means that there is to be no lag in the action). When a motorcycle is firmly tied to the bed of a pickup truck, it will move in real time with the truck. If not, it will lag behind when the truck moves forward from a static position and when it stops.

It is very common for a person to initially counteract by directly resisting a force first before relaxing to make a move, such as contracting the biceps more when feeling a downward pressure, and then easing off this contraction to make a move. This creates the lag in response time. Dan Chisau, when exercised properly, will help to eliminate this problem. The exercise trains you to respond in real time by knowing the value of neutralization and how to achieve this state of equilibrium. The founders of Wing Chun summarized this state of equilibrium and real-time action as Chi (黐), meaning Stickiness. This means having your arm stick to your opponent's as if it was glued there. Whenever or wherever he moves, your arm moves with it in real time. However, it doesn't imply that you stick to your opponent's arm everywhere it goes, but that you do it enough to read and control your opponent's actions.

So, when your partner lowers his wrist and forearm, you must also move your wrist and forearm in the same direction in real time. Although he has some advantage over you because of the opening he has created for an upcoming attack, you have not lost control of the situation because you still have an ongoing forward force pressuring against his to form neutrality. In other words, the situation is still neutral. In a real situation, you could be in a better position in this scenario that appears favorable to him, if you could sense his force but he couldn't sense yours; i.e., you are trained to sense and neutralize a force, but he is not.

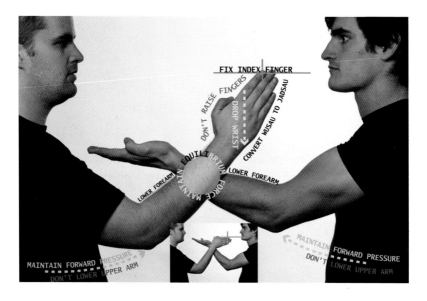

Joe fixes his index finger and drops his wrist, which causes his forearm to lower down—thus, lowering Isaac's forearm; Isaac only allows his forearm to lower down, and keeps his upper arm pressuring forward at the contact point towards Joe's Centerline.

Now that your partner has neutralized your attack and also created an opening, he will carefully execute a punch towards your Centerline. He will do this by converting his open-palm hand to a vertical fist aimed at your Centerline at the same horizontal plane as the prepared fist. Here, he gets to practice how to punch forward and still maintain neutrality in the contact. He will not punch your head just because it appears open for attack, but rather he will punch according to the position of your arm that he is in contact with, and which his force is in equilibrium with. If, for example, his Jadsau was on your wrist or forearm at your solar-plexus height, and he proceeded to punch toward your face, he would then have to leave the neutral contact he had and will no longer "feel" where your arm is and what it is going to do next. Moreover, he will have given up the forward force, at which time, your forward force will no longer have any resistance, thus allowing you to proceed straight forward with a strike, which will have a shorter distance to travel than his upward-traveling punch.

Since he has neutralized your 10 km/h forward Pian Jeong (偏掌—Slant Palm) strike force with his 10 km/h upper arm forward force and steered your arm downward and to the side of the Centerline Plane with his Jadsau, as well as aligned his fist to your Centerline—all in one action—he can now proceed with his attack.

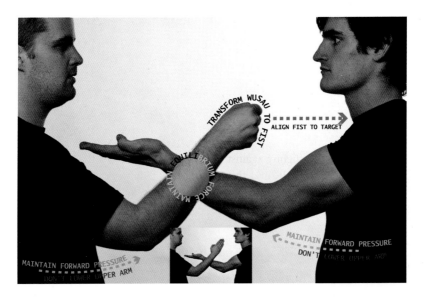

Now that Joe has created an opening with a Jadsau, he forms a fist aimed at Isaac's Centerline; he keeps a check on Isaac's arm by maintaining forward pressure on the contact point; Isaac does the same.

Now—to proceed with the attack, he must now step on his gas pedal to drive his fist at 15 km/h. Since his Jadsau was on the Centerline Plane (that caused your strike to deflect), he must continue the attack on this plane, which means that he must make his forearm travel along the Centerline Plane on the point of contact on your arm. In other words, he will create new points of contact on his own forearm when moving forward, but stay on that one point of contact on your forearm. It is important that he doesn't try to over-control your arm by using his triceps to press down on your arm while punching. If he does this, he will signal his intention too obviously, and also lose the potential to generate full thrusting power, which is taken away by the downward force.

This punching exercise in Dan Chisau is very unique and vitally important to learn. No other martial arts do their punching exercises in this way. For that matter, most Wing Chun practitioners don't do it this way. It is simple in theory, but rather difficult to master. In theory, the arm and hand action of punching is exactly the same as that of using a handsaw to saw through a wooden beam. The upper arm joint and elbow work together in a timely manner to put out the exact amount of force required to saw into the wood little by little. If too much force is put into the action, the saw will get stuck. If the upper arm, forearm, fist, the handle of the saw and the blade from back to front weren't aligned in the same plane, it will lose force, get stuck in the wood, and bend or even break the blade. If the muscles working the rotation of the upper arm and the muscles working the opening and closing of the elbow joint, and the muscles working the wrist don't synchronize properly, or don't direct the bones in the same direction of the force, you will burn more energy than necessary, and also lose force and direction. In sawing, you would begin with the intent of thrusting the blade with a force that will cut 2 millimeters deep (depending on the density of the wood and sharpness of the blade). You would angle the blade slightly against the wood for that. After the first thrust, you would retract the blade, and thrust another 2 millimeters deep; and then repeat the process until completion. However, if you angled the blade more with the intention of thrusting 20 millimeters (2 centimeters) deep right from the start, then you will surely get the blade stuck on your first attempt, which would probably be 2 millimeters deep (this would be the limitation caused by the density of the wood and sharpness of the blade) anyway. Similarly, your punch must travel in the same coordinated manner, aligned in the same manner, and forced in the same manner as cutting wood with a handsaw. Your ulnar bone must cut into the opponent's arm about 2 millimeters deep—just deep enough to feel its presence (place a check on it), and just enough to move it out of the way. This is why it is important to keep your fist in a vertical position so that you can use the edge of your ulna bone to feel and cut the opponent's arm. (You couldn't do that with a horizontally shaped fist—in the supine or pronate position.) Additionally, if the opponent was sensitive enough to detect the cut and either resist or attack you with the same arm, you will be able to neutralize it with the force of your upper arm bone, the humerus, which is directly behind the ulna bone. You couldn't do the same using the flat part of the ulna bone when your fist is turned upward or downward. It would be like trying to saw wood with the flat part of the blade.

You must have an equal amount of cutting force applied onto your opponent's forearm with your forearm contact from front to back when punching along his arm. You must not lift off the front of the forearm at the wrist or from the back (elbow), just as you wouldn't want your car's front or rear tires to lift off when driving. Your constant frontal and rear forearm contact against your opponent's arm when traveling will give you the control that you need over your own arm and his, just as you would with your car when the front and rear tires are always pressed against the road.

Your partner must also make sure that his upper arm, forearm, and fist are aligned in the same plane and traveling path towards your Centerline. The common error is to have a small shoulder abduction, which causes the upper arm (thus the elbow) to slightly swing out sideways away from Centerline. With this poor alignment, your fist will travel forward on the

Centerline Plane, but your forearm and upper arm will travel sideways. To ensure a full and direct hit, you must have the correct alignment, and travel on one point of the opponent's forearm with many of yours rather than many of his with one of yours.

With Tansau, Fooksau, Punching, and other arm-extending actions, the upper arm swings up (forward) and down (backward), pushing and retracting the forearm that is driving the hand/fist on the surface of the opponent's arm. Although the shoulder mechanism allows many other shoulder and upper arm movements, Wing Chun is mainly concerned with the forward (flexion) and backward (extension) movements of the upper arm because of its principle and objective of always driving the arm and hand towards the opponent's Centerline along the Centerline Plane.

Now, as your partner proceeds with his punch along one point of your forearm, and you sense his additional advancing force, you must respond with a forward force from your upper arm to accelerate from 10 km/h to 15 km/h in order to match and neutralize his force. Here again, you must not initiate your action *before* his attack, even though it has become predictable from routine exercises. You must allow him to make some advance before proceeding with the next action.

The next action, without stopping, will have you execute a Bongsau to direct his attack to another direction and out of harm's way.

Here again, you will do the Bongsau correctly, just like you did with your Tansau and Slant-Palm Strike with your partner. You must not abduct your shoulder joint to swing the upper arm laterally sideways away from your Centerline. Lifting your arm against someone pressing or even resting his arm on it will hurt your shoulder when done repeatedly; many Wing Chun practitioners suffer shoulder pain because of this. Bongsau is not a lifting action; it is a corkscrewing action.

The correct way to execute the Bongsau is to first release any tension on your hand—from straight palm and fingers to small curvy palm and fingers, like when you have your arms and hands hanging down the sides doing nothing. Next, you swing your upper arm forward and rotate it laterally (clockwise for the left arm) at the same time, ensuring that you are not swinging the upper arm outside of the shoulder-side parameter, but maintaining the shoulder-joint angle (formed by your humerus and clavicle) the same as you did with the Tansau, Slant-Palm Strike in the last position. In other words, the upper arm keeps moving in the same direction—towards you partner's Centerline—from beginning to end. When done correctly, your shoulder-joint angle will not open wider than 90 degrees or close narrower than 67.5 degrees (90 minus 22.5). When you abduct your shoulder joint, the upper arm will open wider than 90 degrees. What causes most Wing Chun practitioners to erroneously swing their upper arms upward and outward (abduct the shoulder joint) when doing the Bongsau is because they fix their wrist and hand in one vertical plane; they don't move it forward in a corkscrew manner. So, you must continue your forward movement while rotating your upper arm. At the full completion of the upper arm rotation, you then complete the remaining turn of your forearm until the edge of your ulna bone cuts into your partner's ulna bone at 15 km/h, causing a stop to his advance through neutralization.

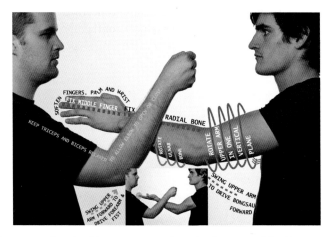

Joe initiates a punch, using his upper arm to drive the forearm and fist; Isaac senses it—so advances and rotates his upper arm first—using his middle finger and radius as the forward-moving axle for ulna rotation.

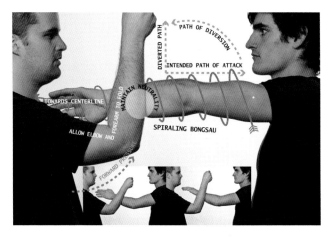

Isaac continues spiraling his arm toward Joe's Centerline, thus rolls Joe's punch away from the intended path; Joe does not resist the path change by locking his elbow, but maintains neutrality where the arms intercept—using upper arm forward pressure.

There are other important things to note about the Bongsau

Firstly, when your partner converted his Fooksau to Jadsau, he took your forearm down and away from the Centerline Plane. However, although your middle finger is no longer pointing towards his Centerline, your elbow is unmoved, and still pointing towards his Centerline. His Jadsau is pressured against your forearm on the Centerline Plane. Therefore, when you perform the Bongsau, you must not push the end of your upper arm towards your middle finger anymore (as in the Siu Nim Tau form), but rather towards his contact point on your forearm and direct it toward his Centerline.

Secondly, the rotation of the Bongsau should not be initiated by the hand or wrist, but by the upper arm for these reasons: The hand or wrist rotation is caused by the radial bone on the forearm rotating around the ulna bone. This action is independent of the humerus. From the upward facing position of your (supinated) palm, you will require to rotate (pronate) the radius 180 degrees before locking the elbow joint to rotate the upper arm to finish the Bongsau. However, if you begin rotating the upper arm from the supinated-palm position, the upper arm will automatically force the radius to rotate. On completion of the upper arm rotation, you will have rotated the radius fully so the edge of the ulna is vertically on top of the radius for the Bongsau position. This is why it is important to relax the hand first to allow the upper arm to rotate the radius fully. This method is more efficient than rotating the hand first because one action or one set of muscles will rotate both the upper arm and forearm; whereas, the other way requires two independent steps and sets of muscles. Moreover, when you have detected an attack coming from a point on your forearm, the attack has already advanced towards you. Reacting with the forearm would be a delayed action because (a) the attacking arm's contact point has already left yours, and (b) the travel distance from that contact point to your brain and back to the point is longer than the point from your brain to the upper arm joint.

So, when performing the Bongsau against your partner's advancing slow-moving punch, you must also do it slowly and consciously, and apply the matching amount of force to deflect and stop further advance.

At this point, it is important to know the design of the human forearm. I will explain it in simple layman terms. The forearm has two long bones; the ulna and the radius. The large end of the ulna fits into an indent of the humerus (upper arm bone) to form the outer elbow joint, and the smaller end terminates at the wrist behind the ring and pinky fingers. It acts as the stabilizing bone from which the radius pivots around. The radius runs parallel to the ulna, with the smaller end fitting into an indent of the humerus to form the inner elbow joint, and the larger end terminating at the wrist behind the thumb, index, and middle finger. The pronator and supinator muscles rotate the radius around the ulna to turn the hand facing down (pronate) or facing up (supinate). The ulna can be made to rotate around the radius by fixing the radius position; however, in actuality, it is still the mechanism of the radius that is rotating around the ulna that makes it appear as if the ulna is rotating around the radius.

So, when you execute the Bongsau, and rotate your upper arm, the forearm will also rotate; i.e., the radius will rotate around the ulna. However, the correct way of doing it is to fix your radial bone contact against his ulna bone contact, and router it out of the Centerline Plane with your ulna, while maintaining the forward advancing force from your upper arm against his contact towards his Centerline. In a fast-paced situation, your opponent's arm will be deflected sideways if it traveled kinetically; however, if he applied compression force against your well-aligned and grounded Bongsau, his arm will deflect upward, which will rock his structure backward if he is not grounded as well as you are.

The two things not to do when executing the Bongsau are to swing the upper arm (from the shoulder joint) trans-medially (toward or across your Centerline) or swing it out (abduct away from the Centerline) trans-laterally.

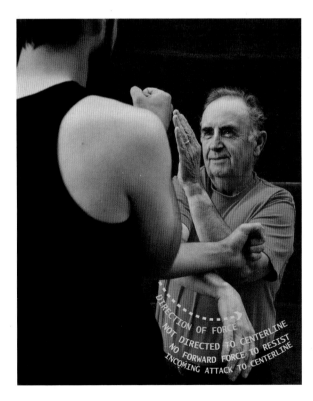

David swings his Bongsau trans-medially; thus, the force is directed away from the Centerline Plane, leaving it unprotected and unpowered.

[173]

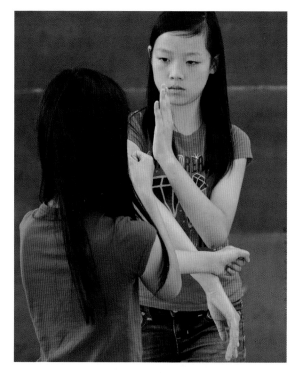

Jade makes the same mistake against Angel's punch.

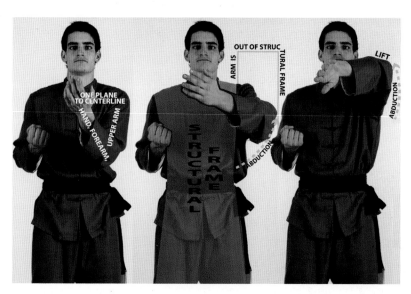

Isaac abducts his shoulder joint, thus lifting his upper arm outside his body frame and diminishing structural support and strength.

[174]

Once you deviate from the 90-degree shoulder-joint angle, you will lose the structural support for the Bongsau. In order to maintain the 90-degree shoulder-joint angle that you began with from the Tansau to the Slant-Palm attack, you must pay attention to circle your elbow around the axis located between your outer and inner elbow, and that the axis must not travel outside of the original upper arm alignment of approximately 90 degrees against the chest. It can travel upward or downward—and still maintain the 90 degree angle—but not travel sideways. If that sounds complicated, it is not. When a gun is aimed at a target, and the bullet is fired, it travels on one vertical plane—determined by the alignment of the gun barrel towards the target; the bullet spins around its own singular axis. The gun could point upward or downward; nonetheless, the bullet will still travel straight on one vertical plane at an incline or decline, and spin around its own axis. It will not sway sideways unless the barrel or bullet is poorly crafted. So, similarly, the Bongsau can travel upward or downward, but the upper arm will rotate on one axis along the one vertical plane. The axis should not swing nor travel sideways to anywhere outside of the one vertical plane.

Note that the height of the Bongsau will vary depending on the difference between your height and that of your partner's, and also on the height of his attack. As mentioned before, you must not leave a contact point to execute an attack. A Bongsau, in essence, is an attack. You are advancing towards his Centerline, with the intent of destroying his structure in the process. Therefore, the height of your Bongsau will depend on the height of his punch. If it were in the middle zone, you would direct the force to the middle; if it were in the middle-low zone, you would direct the force at a decline; and if it were in the high zone, you would direct the force at an incline.

The properties of the Middle and Low Bongsau are somewhat different from a High Bongsau. For a Middle or Middle-Low Bongsau, the shoulder is always higher than the elbow; the elbow is higher than the wrist; and the wrist is higher than the fingers. In other words, the arm and hand declines from the shoulder. For the High Bongsau, the rule reverses; i.e. the fingers are now higher than the wrist; the wrist is higher than the elbow; and the elbow is higher than the shoulder. In other words, the arm and hand inclines from the shoulder. When you think about it, it makes good sense why the properties change for different heights. In order to always project an advancing force towards your opponent's Centerline you must direct your upper arm's force to your opponent's Centerline through your fingertips (particularly the middle finger). Therefore, your fingers should always be pointing at a spot on it. They shouldn't be pointing beyond any physical spot such as above the opponent's head, below his crotch or outside his shoulders' parameters. (This principle applies to all other Wing Chun "hands.") You should never do a High Bongsau where your elbow is higher than the shoulders, but the wrist and fingers are below the elbow. Although you may have your fingers pointing at the opponent's Centerline, your elbow will be pointing upwards instead, thus, you will no longer have the required advancing force from the upper arm towards your opponent's Centerline.

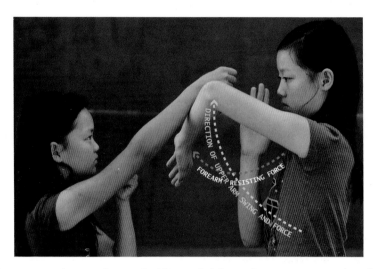

Jade executes an incorrect Bongsau by lifting and abducting her upper arm trans-laterally to deflect Angel's punch, however, her force is upward rather than forward, and will not stop a structural advance, but topple her backward.

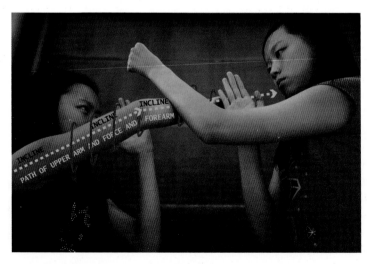

Angel executes a correct Bongsau by spiraling her arm at an incline toward Jade's Centerline; it has forward, resisting, and deflecting force.

When you execute the Bongsau to neutralize your partner's punch in the Dan Chisau exercise, your partner must not apply more than the 15 km/h forces that he initiated. He must not press down on your Bongsau, forcefully push his punch forward, or forcefully steer back his deflected arm to the Centerline Plane. He must let you deflect and neutralize his force, yet have control over his own force and yours in the equilibrium state. This can only be done if he puts out just the right amount of force— no more and no less—than what is required, and that he is fully aware of every moment of the contact and process of the punch. He must also always keep his elbow vertically below the interception point (the contact point where his forearm meets yours) so that his forearm can act as a vertical obstacle against any attack coming towards his Centerline from below the contact point by either the opponent's contacted arm or the free arm. Practitioners tend to stretch their arms fully, wanting to hit a physical target with their punch. For one, the Dan Chisau is not a point-scoring competition. Secondly, even in a real fight, hitting a target at arm's length with a fully stretched arm—when the punch has come to the end of its maximum distance and energy—will barely have any penetrating force or impact. It would be like standing above a barrel of dry beans at arm's length, and punching into it just one-inch deep. You need to be close enough to the target, when the elbow is still bent, to hit it with a driving force that will allow you to penetrate your arm elbow deep. In order to deliver such a penetrating punch in a real situation when the opponent is at arm's length, you would need to bridge the distance by stepping into his zone, instead of just staying static structurally and stretching your arm to hit the target.

As mentioned earlier, a fully-opened elbow will rise up and open the gates for the opponent to attack your Centerline under your arm. Although trying to remember and follow all these precautionary safety rules may appear to be a slow process for a real, fast fighting situation, it won't be so when you have made it into a second-nature habit as a result of training regularly for a long time. The more you train, the less you need to think about them; your brain will respond faster and more accurately to these rules the more you practice. It is no different than driving. When you first learned to drive, there seemed to be too many details to remember. You were required to train your limbs to coordinate them with the controls of the car plus watch the road, traffic, and other drivers while you were driving. After months and years, however, you didn't need to think about them anymore, and your brain was able to handle all the details, plus add more such as listening to music, having a conversation, and chewing on a burger at the same time.

Finally, for the Chisau exercise, the two of you will return to the original equilibrium state of 5 km/h force against each other by you initiating the conversion of Bongsau to Tansau, and your opponent converting his fist to a Fooksau. You must rotate your Bong arm and release the force (pressure on the gas pedal) slowly and incrementally from 15 km/h pressure down to 5 km/h pressure. He must also follow your arm action by slowly and incrementally releasing and matching your force while converting the fist hand to Fooksau. Both of you must return to the 5 km/h force from the 15 km/h force in the neutral state all the way from start to finish. When you convert and reduce your 15 km/h Bongsau to the 5 km/h Tansau, you must not drop your Tan hand vertically down like many practitioners do. That will open the path for your opponent to strike your Centerline above your arm. You must retract the hand along the same path that it originally inclined. You will therefore decline on that path from 15 km/h to 5 km/h. This will allow you to drive your arm up at an incline again if your opponent changes direction and attacks you, at which point your upward driving Tansau will neutralize and/or deflect it; or, you can attack your opponent's Centerline if you felt that his force has dropped below yours, thus, causing an imbalanced force (no longer in the equilibrium state). If you had dropped down your Tansau vertically instead of retracting it at a decline, you will no longer have the pushing power of your upper arm or forearm, but will be left with very little lifting power against your opponent's arm force above it, which is additionally supported by gravity's force. If you had to do the Bongsau after this, you'd have to lift it upward instead of thrusting it like a corkscrew, which is much easier than a lifting it from a dead hang.

So, in the exercise, as you will recoil your Bongsau to Tansau, and your partner must also retract his fist and convert it to Fooksau in time with your movement until both of your wrists meet at the original starting point of the exercise. This will bring the Dan Chisau cycle to completion. That doesn't mean that you have finished the exercise, but that you will begin the cycle again, and do it repeatedly every training session until you and your sifu are satisfied that you've achieved some degree of mastery over it.

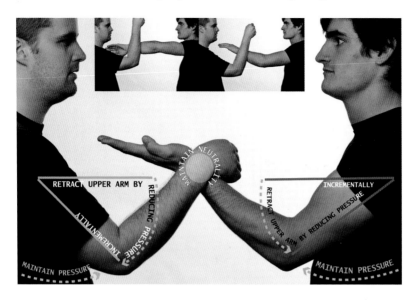

Isaac initiates a return to the original position by reducing the forward pressure of his upper arm incrementally while spiraling his arm backward—transforming Bongsau to Tansau; Joe matches Isaac's reducing force by retracting his upper arm—transforming the fist to Fooksau.

The Dan Chisau exercise can be diversified by changing roles such as you doing the Fooksau part and your partner doing the Tansau part, and then doing the cycle with your other arms. You can also attack the partner's chest (instead of the throat) with an Upright-Palm strike from the Tansau position, or attack your partner's ribs with a Low Slant-Palm strike. Each action will need to be tweaked using the same concept of neutralization and diversion.

The Dan Chisau, apart from teaching a student the proper use of Tansau, Slant-Palm Strike, Fooksau, Jadsau, Sun-Character Punch and Bongsau, also teaches you to read force, respond with neutrality, and apply force from the upper arm, support your upper arm force with your square structure and ground, always drive your force towards your opponent's Centerline relentlessly, use the wrist to steer the hand and forearm, attack with defense in mind, and defend with attack in mind.

Another very important lesson in the Dan Chisau exercise is the affirmation of the upper arm usage for force, which is already taught and exercised in the Siu Nim Tao form.

THE MYTH OF ELBOW POWER

Wing Chun practitioners talk a lot about elbow power, but in reality the elbow is a very weak joint articulated by the biceps and triceps of the upper arm, which are relatively small muscles compared to other muscles on the body. It is susceptible to inescapable arm locks, such as the arm-bar that grapplers love to use.

The elbow joint is weak because of its design, for both flexing and extending. It is designed for mobility, not stability. There is always a tradeoff between mobility and stability. As you may recall from the chapter on structure, when you design something very mobile, then you will have little stability; conversely, if you design something very stable, then it will have little mobility.

The human structure is made up of bones, which are held together and moved by ligaments, tendons and muscles. The bones act as levers; the joints, made from two or more bones, which are attached by ligaments act as fulcrums, while the muscles, which are attached to the bones by tendons, serve as the force that moves the bones. In other words, the human structure is made up of a bunch of moving levers.

There are three classes of levers. A lever (linear or circular) will have a fulcrum (a fixed point), a load (or weight), and a force (or effort) to act on it. A Class-1 Lever has the fulcrum between the force and load. Examples of simple machines with Lever-1 classification would be seesaws, wire cutters and pliers. Class-2 lever have the fulcrum at one end of the lever, and the force will be applied at the other end of the lever, while the load will be placed between the fulcrum and the effort end. Examples of Class-2 levers would be wheelbarrows, nutcrackers and bottle openers. To obtain a mechanical advantage from these levers, the effort/force arm must be longer than the load arm. The ratio between the two will proportionately increase or decrease the mechanical advantage. Class-3 levers will have the fulcrum at one end of the lever, the load at the other end of the lever, and the force will be applied between the two. This type of lever has absolutely no mechanical advantage, no matter where you move the load or effort along the lever. Although a longer effort arm will provide a greater advantage over a shorter one, it will not multiply the input force to a higher output force. The only time that you will get an equal amount of output force from the input force is if the effort is applied directly onto the load. In that case, however, you wouldn't need a lever. You could just push or lift the load with your hands without it. Examples of Class-3 levers would be tweezers, chopsticks and brooms. They're only good for light and small work.

When you flex your arm (bending the elbow), you are performing a Class-3 Lever action, with absolutely no mechanical advantage. Your biceps are attached to an insertion point on your forearm bone just in front of the elbow fulcrum. By design, it is not only weak because of being a Class-3 Lever design, i.e., the fulcrum is at one end and the load at the other end (e.g., a weight on the hand), but the effort arm is extremely short compared to the load arm.

When you open your elbows and extend your arm, you are performing a Class-1 Lever action. Because the elbow doesn't allow you to fold your arm all the way to the back of the upper arm, but only to a straightened position, the triceps needn't attach to the forearm in front of the elbow like the biceps do; instead, it is attached to the upper end of the ulna forearm bone—slightly behind the elbow joint. Although a Class-1 Lever by design will have more mechanical advantage than Class-3 lever, in this case it will not because of the shortness of the effort arm; i.e., from insertion point to fulcrum. So now that we know that the elbow mechanism cannot generate much in the way of power, what are the Wing Chun people talking about? Most of them don't know what they're talking about. They're just parroting what they've heard from their sifus.

In Wing Chun the true role of the elbow is to serve as a reference point. It is referencing the upper arm—the use of the upper arm instead of the elbow mechanism. The elbow is at the end of the upper arm. When you move the upper arm, you move the elbow point. Flexing or extending the upper arm will render a much stronger force than flexing or extending the forearm. The upper arm bone, the humerus, is moved by a network of large muscles in the chest, shoulder and back. The insertions are attached to the head of the bone at the shoulder joint or a little way down the shaft, allowing a variety of movements. At first look, the design—short effort arm—might appear to be mechanically disadvantageous; however, after careful examination, you will see why it can render tremendous power. First, the muscles associated with it are multiple, large, and linked to other muscles in the front and back. It would be like having 20 strong men using a long chain to pull a heavy rock instead of three men pulling with a short rope (as in the case of triceps usage). Moreover, the back muscles are indirectly or directly attached to the spine, which of course, is the nucleus of the body frame. From this connection, these muscles can tap other large muscles for use such as the muscles on the pelvis and legs.

Although the elbow mechanism has no mechanical advantage, it does have the advantage of speed and distance coverage. For example, if the fulcrum was placed one meter from the effort point of a four meter lever, making the effort arm one meter long and the load arm three meters long, then for every 10 centimeters the effort arm is lowered, the end of the load arm will travel 30 centimeters or three times higher; thus, covering more distance. It also means that if it took 1/100th of a second to move 10 centimeters of the effort arm, the load arm traveled three times that distance in the same amount of time, thus, rendering speed advantage.

The elbow, therefore, should be used as a reference point in the use of the upper arm, particularly in aligning the forearm and hand to it when traveling toward the opponent's centerline; whether for striking, resisting, or deflecting an incoming force. Furthermore, the elbow should be aligned to the pelvic point, knee and heel of the powering side of the body. On the other hand, the forearm and hand, beyond the elbow, should only be used as a projectile or the load of the upper arm lever instead of a power tool. Don't use the biceps and triceps—the elbow mechanism—for delivering or resisting force, but use it to maximize speed and distance.

COMPRESSION AND TENSION FORCES

Apart from dealing with kinetic forces from (or using them against) your opponent, you will also need to deal with compression and tension forces. By definition, compression results from forces acting towards each other; whereas, tension results from forces acting away from each other. In other words, compression pushes things together, and tension pulls things apart.

You can only make your muscles contract; you cannot stretch them from a static position without contracting some other antagonist (or opposing) muscles. They will only stretch upon relaxing them and allowing the antagonist muscles to pull the bones associated with them. However, by contracting them, you can make the joints open or close to move the bones forward or backward for pushing or pulling actions.

In the Paksau drills, you learn to develop and deliver powerful kinetic energy. You throw a punch by contracting and immediately releasing the muscles associated with the punching action. Your partner reacts similarly with a Paksau, Tansau, Lapsau (拉手—Pulling Arm), or whatever. However, punching and neutralizing is not all there is to fighting; you will end up fighting your opponent using both compression and tension forces by resisting his pull or push. You can train and develop compressional and tensional forces in the Dan Chisau, Seung Chisau, or trapping exercises by applying more pressure than the minimum exercised in the beginning. However, you don't want to end up merely rocking each other back and forth. There are other, better two-man exercises to develop compressional and tensional awareness and strength, but the best one is working on the Wooden-Man Post (木人樁)—also referred to as the dummy.

[182]

TRAINING ON THE WOODEN DUMMY

Here again, many practitioners make the mistake of using the dummy to slap and move around it quickly. They build the dummy torso very light, the frame springy, and the arms wobbly to accomplish that. Unfortunately, all they get out of it are loud noises and self-aggrandizement.

Western sports are normally based on physical speed and strength, as evident in the Olympic Games. This is not to say that skills are not involved, but these skills are quite different from what is required to excel in the Asian martial arts, both in terms of concepts and goals. Many Western sports involve running, and therefore require the athletes to have light legs and a lot of stamina for greater endurance; whereas, martial artists require large legs for balance and grounding, and conserved energy for intermittent explosive usage. For physical exercises, Westerners tend to build large muscles on their shoulders, arms, and chests and like to have tight "6-pack" stomach muscles; whereas, martial artists are required to have soft shoulders and arms for mobility and a soft waist for storing large amounts of energy.

Wing Chun practitioners who grow up with Western sports tend to emphasize speed and upper body strength, and, thus, when working the dummy tend to gravitate towards performance style of training on it, which consists of slapping the dummy's arms and torso quickly, and shuffling around it on the balls of their feet as quickly as possible. That's not what the dummy was designed for. Moreover, if your goal is to practice and enhance explosive kinetic energy and footwork, there are other exercises—such as striking a wall bag or walking on lines that will accomplish this more effectively. Think about it logically, the dummy is made out of wood—you can't punch it with full force, otherwise you would break your wrist or another bone—even if you placed padding on it. This is why many practitioners slap it—but that is not what it is for either. Also, the dummy is stationary. Your opponent will not be. You can't possibly walk around your opponent as you can with the dummy. Your opponent is never going to be that dumb and slow. All of the sifus who demo the walk-around dummy technique with a cooperating partner are in denial. They should know better because they can't even do it when they spar with their students, unless the students are really unskilled or super cooperative. If they try to walk around a boxer, they'll get clipped with a hook that will reset their jaws. If it were so easy to do, boxers would be doing that in the ring already.

In the dummy form, you are forced to walk around to the side of the dummy *because it is stationary*. In reality, you only make that step-in attack if you are able to turn your opponent to expose his side, or if he has turned himself to expose it.

The dummy was designed for you to develop compressional and tensional force. The force is driven by your pelvic muscles and legs to the ground and delivered upward to your arms as I described earlier in some detail regarding the mechanics of the explosive punch, but it is done with compression or tension upon contact. Many practitioners leave the contact they've established in one movement of the dummy and reconnect to it with another, which is not wrong, but does not give them the compressional and tensional exercise they need in addition to the kinetic exercises they've received in other training. By leaving a contact point and stepping into the dummy to establish a new contact point, they are using their body's kinetic force to bang into it. That is something you may need to do to initially to bridge into an opponent's space; however, what do you when you've bridged and not succeeded in finishing off the opponent? (The likelihood of not finishing him off in one movement is much higher than finishing him with just one movement by the way.) Do you leave that contact and reconnect with another attack? If you do, you are no longer connected with him so you won't know his next move or the amount of incoming force. On the other hand, if you do not leave the contact and have established neutrality, you are able to respond more effectively. If he increases his force against you, you can increase yours accordingly. So, if you've trained yourself to counter a massive force, whether it is compressional or tensional, you will then not only be able to resist it, but overpower it. If you've trained yourself to deliver the force from your pelvis to the ground to your arms, and your opponent has not, he will bounce off your force.

Compressional and tensional forces are different than kinetic force. With kinetic force, such as a punch, it will travel and meet your kinetic force, such as a Paksau, with a sudden impact. With compression and tension, two forces begin from "0" or a state of equilibrium, and increase incrementally. They may increase quickly or slowly, but nonetheless, they increase incrementally rather than coming into forcible contact. Two cars crashing head-on into each other creates an impact from their kinetic forces; whereas, when two cars are crushed by a compactor in the recycle yard, they are flattened by compression force. Boxers hit each other with kinetic-thrown punches, but wrestlers use compression and tension force to put each other down or into locks. As seen in the ring, sluggers fail miserably against good grapplers, and grapplers fail miserably against good sluggers. However, Wing Chun competitors fail miserably against both because most of them can't punch with kinetic force and fewer still have developed compressional or tensional strength.

If you want to be as well-rounded a Wing Chun practitioner as possible, then you must train to develop compressional or tensional strength.

You need to have a heavy dummy to train on, and you need to hang it on a heavy freestanding structure, allowing little give in the arms and torso of the dummy. When doing the dummy form (the only apparatus form in Wing Chun), don't leave a contact point once you've established it—at least have one contact point established when changing from one movement to another, and only leave it when another contact point has been established. When walking around the dummy, use one contact point as the fulcrum to move around it and always maintain a neutral force on a contact point before increasing it—do not hop in, out, and around the dummy but move your feet flat on the ground. Use the sagittal side of your defensive hand such as the Tansau to deliver compressional force against the dummy's centerline through the arm that your Tansau is pressing against, and use your free side to deliver a kinetic strike to the dummy's torso. Execute all of your kinetic strikes from close range. Most of the Gangsau (耕手—Plowing Arm) and Gwansau (滾手—Rolling Arms) should be performed compressionally, and all pulling actions should be done tensively. All Baopai (抱派—Carrying the Signage) or Popai (破派—Splitting the Signage) actions should be done with a mixture of compression and kinetic forces; i.e., first connect your hands to the dummy compressionally and then deliver an explosive force (because they are not strikes, but rather, powerful pushes); and all leg connection to the dummy's leg must be done compressionally except for kicks. These are just some pointers on how to train to better develop compression and tension strength on the dummy.

The reason I recommend a freestanding dummy on a heavy frame rather than on a wall-mounted dummy is because you can move the dummy back with your compressional force when you push or strike at it during the performance of the form. Additionally, you can practice strike-pushing it with combined compressional and kinetic forces with the linear quarter-step footwork that you've learned in the Chum Kiu form. (You can also develop strong lower-trunk compressional and tensional strength by having a partner resist your quarter-step or full walk by pushing against your two pelvic sides in front of you or pulling at them from the back while you walk linearly).

I always remind myself that this is an art developed by women, and that the training program must be executed with this in mind. The training cannot be so taxing that a woman or a man of small stature cannot do it, but something realistic that a person can do relative to his or her size. The first part of Wing Chun training is to make that person first find and express his or her full potential based on the laws of physics, biomechanics and DNA—whether the person is a male or female, tall or short, fat or skinny, young or old. Once this is established, the person can choose to optimize or more fully realize his potential by building stronger muscles and/or stamina outside of the Wing Chun training curriculum. The Wing Chun training program was designed for fight-or-flight situations, meaning that the muscles and mind are to be trained for sudden intensive actions rather than regular rhythmic actions such as jogging or swimming. The Wing Chun forms and drills were designed to develop the muscles and mind to deal with aggressive kinetic, compressional, and tensional forces, which is what happens when a real fight ensues.

In the Siu Nim Tao form we learn movements that can be performed kinetically as well as compressionally and tensionally. I teach my students to perform them very slowly to develop the muscles required to deal with compressional and tensional forces. At completion of the form, I have them do all the moves again—only this time explosively from Section Two onwards. From Chum Kiu onwards, the forms teach us to use our pelvis to deliver a torque force to enhance our kinetic, compressional and/or tensional force.

So, in reality, the Wing Chun program is designed to deal with sluggers, grapplers, and wrestlers. The reason why Wing Chun practitioners have often failed against them is because they have not understood the philosophies, goals, or the training program that the creators of Wing Chun originally outlined for them. In addition, many fail simply because they're not willing to put in the time necessary to study and train like other competitors and martial artists. Sadly, the primary reason most do not develop fully in this art is that their egos prevent them from learning all that there is to know and opening themselves up to becoming great in the art.

TWELVE

Speed: The Science of Time and Space

MANY PEOPLE HAVE THE notion that speed is the most important factor in fighting. However, the reality is that the speed from one person to another does not vary much, especially in punching. A punching fist travels no more than a meter from a fully cocked position until it hits its target. At that speed, how much of a difference could there be from the fastest puncher in the world to the slowest?

I recall once reading in M. Nakayama's book *Dynamic Karate*, which was published in 1966, that they had used a stroboscope with a flash time of 1/10,000 of a second to measure the punch of a Karateka. The stroboscope indicated that the Karateka's punch was measured at a speed of 43 feet/second, generating an impact power equal to 1,500 pounds. Let us imagine for the moment that this impressive feat has been exceeded, and that the fastest puncher now punches three times as fast (i.e., 129 feet/second). If the two record holders from the past and present stood in front of each other one meter apart with their fists cocked back, and fired their punches at each other's chests at the same time, do you think you would hear two distinctive thuds, one after the other? If you think so, let me give you another example to consider.

If an old 1966 Volkswagen (VW) Beetle can max out at 70 mph, and sprint from 0 to 40 mph in 8.5 seconds, and a 2014 Ferrari can max out at 210 mph (three times the speed of VW), and sprint from 0 to 120 mph in 8.5 second (three times the acceleration of the VW), and two drivers of equal weight stepped on the gas pedal at the same time from the starting line, how much difference do you think the Ferrari will lead the VW at three feet from the starting line? Will it be noticeable to the naked eye? I don't think so. Could the difference be captured by a super-speed camera? Maybe, but how much would it be? My guess is less than ⅛ inch.

The reality is that there is not much difference in the speed of one puncher from another. That is not to say that there is no advantage in delivering a faster punch than your opponent since the more velocity you can generate, the more powerful your punch will be. However, when it comes to measuring the *time* difference between your punch and that of your opponent, the difference is too miniscule to matter. However, if one of the martial artists threw his punch before the other, even by one-tenth of a second, then the difference will become evident. That also goes for the driver who steps on the gas pedal before the other. So, as you can see, it is the timing factor that becomes crucial here rather than the speed factor.

One of Wing Chun's training programs is to condition the practitioner to minimize his pre-firing actions; that is, not to cock his fist before firing a punch. In Wing Chun, it doesn't matter who draws his gun first, but who fires first. If your opponent makes unnecessary moves, such as screaming, bulging his eyes, foaming at the mouth, and winding his fist back to punch, and you don't do the same, but fire your punch from wherever your fist is at, then you will most likely beat him to the punch. Besides the visual detection, Wing Chun's Chisau exercise trains you to feel the opponent's tension and intention through contact, giving you that extra edge.

Now, if you are able to detect an incoming attack, then why just block it with one arm, and follow it with a counter-strike when you can deflect it with one while simultaneously employing the other to strike? I realize that this is easier said than done, however, that's precisely what Chisau training conditions you for. The double arm action of Chisau will save you time, which equates to efficiency and speed. So, instead of executing two separate actions in half a second, you could do the two simultaneously in one quarter of a second. For that matter, why not kick your opponent at the same time? Then you will accomplish three tasks within that same time span. Stated another way; the strategy is: If you send one ruffian to attack me, I will send three of mine to deal with him. In that case, the odds of my success would be much greater than yours!

For the same reason that Wing Chun does not encourage singular punching, it also does not encourage singular kicking; that is, to kick the opponent from a distance that isn't within reach. The reason being that the more distance a kick needs to travel, the more effort and time is required for it to reach the intended target, thus, burning your energy quickly and allowing time for your opponent to react. Additionally, the farther you are away from your opponent, the more visible the kick will be to him, thus, allowing him to anticipate its arrival and better his chances of countering it. Also, should your opponent step back out of the range of your kick, your attempted kick now needs to travel even further than before, with the result that any opportunity for you to apply a three-limb simultaneous attack is now gone. And, if he decides to step into your zone, your kick will have overshot its mark, now allowing him to attack you with his two or three limbs or otherwise imbalance you, as you now are standing on just one leg.

Wing Chun's safety rule states that you must only kick the opponent when you have at least one contact point established from one of your arms that has connected to some part of your opponent. In essence, you will borrow his two grounded legs to form a tripod with your standing leg. For that matter, even if your opponent is on one leg (the other being used to kick or deflect your kick), your arm connection to him will still give you two feet (his one and your one) on the ground. Your arm connection needn't be strong; just a light touch will do. You can test this theorem by standing on one foot beside a wall and touching it with just one fingertip (a wall is a grounded structure.) You will see that you can hold your balance as long as your muscles can endure. On the other hand, without the connection to the wall, you will lose your balance easily.

Wing Chun's kick is often referred to as the Under-the-Skirt kick, meaning that you are so close to the opponent that your kick will be concealed by your skirt. That is not hard to imagine for a girl; however, that also applies to men. In the old days, Chinese men wore long ankle-length gowns as seen attired by Great-Grandmaster Ip Man in some photographs. They were quite close fitting—not frock-like. The gowns had two side slits that allowed freer leg movements such as climbing stairs. The Under-the-Skirt term expresses how close you need to be to your opponent to throw a kick. That close range also allows you to apply your entire arsenal of your fists, palms, forearms, elbows, knees, calves, heels, shoulders, pelvis, and even your head and teeth (if absolutely necessary and effective)—all within reach, and all available to be applied simultaneously in groups of twos and threes.

Wing Chun's leg training is powerful, but only in unison with the other limbs. It does not specialize in kicking as other arts such as Taekwondo or Muay Thai. On a one-to-one comparison for kicking ability and power, Wing Chun will lose to the other two arts. However, the Wing Chun legwork has more functions than just kicking, such as protecting the area below the groin and controlling, trapping, grappling, stomping, and sweeping the opponent's legs or feet. The Wing Chun creators went for quantity instead of quality for the kicks. However, that doesn't mean that the kicks are ineffective, but rather that they were given multiple functions to deal with multiple situations rather than a few strong usages for limited situations. Again, referring to whom Wing Chun was primarily designed for—the person of smaller stature—his or her strong kick may not be so effective against a person with large bones padded with lots of muscles. So, the Wing Chun kick wasn't designed to kick the stomach, chest or head like the kicks employed in other systems, but to kick the most vulnerable areas, such as the knees (particularly the sides and back), the shins, ankles, insteps and toes—all very weak areas of the body, even on very large men. Once you damage or hurt any part of your opponent's leg—the muscles, bones or joints, which your opponent needs and relies on to support his weight and movements—he becomes almost dysfunctional if not disabled. A close-range kick, although lacking momentum force can be powerful because of its weight-bearing property; that is, you are able to apply your weight onto the opponent's leg or feet from that distance and because the angle of attack is narrower than a long kick and, thus, closer to the perpendicular line of gravity, you will require less effort, and even get the support of gravity's force to generate more power for a downward-angled kick.

So, what you saw in the movie, *The Grandmasters*, where the Ip Man character throws high and long roundhouse, front and sidekicks are not within the principles of Wing Chun philosophy. They're more like Taekwondo's. This is not to say that high, long, and strong kicks are ineffective, but that they go against the principles of Wing Chun, and that the movie represents Wing Chun and Ip Man in a poor and untruthful manner in terms of the techniques of his art.

All of the principles of Wing Chun flow from its main concept. Some say that the Wing Chun concept is Close-Range Fighting; however, that doesn't accurately describe the fullness of the Wing Chun concept.

Close-range fighting is not a concept but rather a characteristic derived from the Wing Chun concept. Using the arms and other body parts such as the shoulders, the hips and legs to read the opponent is Wing Chun's concept and strategy. In order to do this, one automatically needs to be at close-range. Other benefits follow from this, such as the ability to use three limbs simultaneously to attack and defend, and the ability to use one's entire arsenal.

Another advantage of training for close-range fighting is that it is the better of two extremes. The other extremity is keeping a considerable distance from your opponent; however, you don't really need special training for that. Soldiers don't need to be taught how to retreat. It is a natural human instinct. The difficult part is to train them to keep advancing when under fire—and so it is likewise in Wing Chun.

If you have the luxury of an area the size of a football field to fight your opponent on, then you can keep him chasing you endlessly. Even in a boxing ring, you can run and dodge your opponent's attacks for twelve rounds if you don't intend to get hit or intend to hit him. So, keeping a safe distance from your opponent is not rocket science; however, fighting close-range is. If you can fight inside an elevator, then you can fight anywhere.

In the animal world, the first thing that one animal does to another when fighting is to attempt to unbalance its prey and take it to the ground. It is a very instinctive action even with humans. Being on the ground is a very vulnerable position. For this reason, Chinese martial arts stress stability very strongly. There are many Chinese and Japanese martial arts that specialize in takedowns and ground fighting such as seen in Mixed Martial Arts (MMA). And there are those who believe that Wing Chun would not fare well against the tactics of MMA. I must confess, after seeing the way that some Wing Chun practitioners train and act, this doesn't surprise me. In fact, many Wing Chun practitioners have gone up against MMA fighters and ended up being tied up in knots. This is not because of the weakness of the Wing Chun concept or its training methods, but rather the result of practitioners who have never really understood the full concept of Wing Chun nor received proper training in the art. However, if they understood and trained according to the true concept and methods outlined by the system, they would not only stand a chance against MMA fighters, but also overcome them easily.

To conclude this chapter, we've looked at speed from the overall perspective of time and space rather than just a person's ability to move his limbs faster than another person. Therefore, speed can be achieved from higher consciousness; i.e. being aware of everything around you, reading your opponent's intent and action, reacting without hesitation or unnecessary moves, using the correct muscles and relaxing the opposing ones, applying just the right amount of intent, energy and force, positioning yourself at the optimum distance and applying the most economical, efficient and productive movement. All of these are brain functions. Being able to accomplish them successfully means that you've trained your brain to engage its sensors and neural machinery more efficiently and effectively. And *that* is what the Wing Chun training program is designed for.

THIRTEEN

Wing Chun: The Science of the Human Body and the Human Mind

Wing Chun's history and concept is very rich and very deep. It would take a lifetime to unravel it and fully comprehend its totality. Nevertheless, the time and effort spent in its unraveling and comprehension is a large part of the beauty and joy of it.

Wing Chun wasn't designed for exhibitions, showmanship, or ego building. It was designed for each individual student's appreciation, and for successful use in a (hopefully) but once-in-a-lifetime life-threatening situation, when you need to bring out your entire arsenal to swiftly and completely destroy an assailant. It wasn't designed for engaging in friendly matches between buddies, nor to play about in a boxing ring with gloves and protective gear, and it certainly wasn't the intent of the founders to feature it in spectacular action movies.

When you spar with a partner in Wing Chun, the sparring should look graceful and beautiful. The two of you should look like you are ballroom dancing; your bodies well composed, connected with each other, moving in unison, and dancing without missing a beat like Fred Astaire and Ginger Rogers. Your faces should not be all tensed up, your bodies should not be taut, and your movements should not be jerky—but that's sparring. When you get into a real fight, it is another ball game entirely. Survival becomes your top priority. You may not be able to perform perfectly like you did with your training partner, and neither will your opponent. However, what will immediately become obvious is the success of the type of training you both have received. If your opponent was trained only to react to certain types of attacks within a certain type of environment, and if his training doesn't match the current situation (which will always be the case because every opponent and environment will be different), then your opponent will be at a disadvantage because he will have trouble adjusting on the fly to the unknown. However, if you've been trained mentally to understand that every opponent and environment will be different, that fighting is the art of managing both force and environment, and if your training involved interactive sparring rather than unrealistic choreographed reaction to situation-based scenarios, then you will have a much better chance of not only surviving, but defeating your opponent. The Wing Chun concept and training program is essentially the laws of physics and biomechanics made applicable to fighting. The principles are not restrictive but are used as guidelines to give the practitioner the best results in terms of safety and performance. In some ways it is no different than training someone to drive a car. The traffic laws are designed for optimum safety and performance for all drivers. You are trained to drive within your lane's parameters, and to watch out for other drivers' movements. If a driver from the opposite side veers into your lane, you don't stay in your lane just because the rules say you should; instead you would swing into the safest lane, even if it were momentarily toward oncoming traffic, just to get out of harm's way. Similarly, you learn and follow safety and performance rules in Wing Chun training. However, in a real fight, you will do whatever it takes to get out of harm's way and perform optimally. You may jump, throw a hook punch, bite or pull your opponent's hair (which is not part of Wing Chun's technical training curriculum, per se), but you will do it automatically because of your inherent desire to survive. These are reflex actions that Wing Chun's training program encourages, rather than represses.

Because Wing Chun's training program is geared toward the natural laws of physics and biomechanics, it will allow you to quickly improvise the tools you've acquired from your training to adapt to any unpredictable and immediate situation. Musashi, in his most well-known duel with Sasaki Kojiro (a man who proved to be his most formidable opponent), extemporaneously carved a wooden oar into a boken or wooden sword while he was on his way to the duel in a boat. He used it to kill his challenger, who wielded a sword made of steel by Japan's finest swordsmith.

Once you understand the Wing Chun concept of fighting, you can fight empty handed, with weapons or without weapons, or against one or multiple opponents. The concept remains the same. You will automatically assess the situation and react appropriately, rather than search your memory bank for pre-rehearsed scenarios that might be suitable for the situation you have now found yourself in. Musashi wrote:

> The spirit of defeating a man is the same as ten million men. If one man can beat ten, then a thousand can beat ten thousand. If you become a master of strategy by training alone with a sword and you understand the enemy's strategies, his strength, and resources, you can apply the strategy to beat ten thousand enemies.

Sadly, many Wing Chun schools have veered away from its traditional training program. Many sifus have previously trained in other systems and therefore feel more comfortable when they infuse their old training programs into the Wing Chun program. Examples of this are when a Wing Chun class performs thirty minutes of warm-ups and calisthenics, forty to sixty minutes of choreographed attack-and-defend drills, and then ten minutes of loosening-up or "cooling down" exercises at the end of the class. None of these were ever a part of any traditional Wing Chun training program and yet a hundred minutes are spent on them out of a two-hour class, leaving only twenty minutes dedicated to actual Wing Chun–related training such as the forms, Chisau, and sparring. Many schools run ninety-minute classes in which they feature lots of fitness exercises by reducing the actual amount of Wing Chun training. When I attended Wing Chun classes in my early years they were never under three hours in length and the senior students spent virtually all of those three hours working on their Chisau and sparring, which trained them in strategy and better understanding their opponents, while the beginners spent more time working on the Wing Chun forms and Paksao drills in order to develop and strengthen their fundamental understanding of the Wing Chun concept of fighting. This is how I conduct my classes still.

Wing Chun is so deep that you need a lot of time to train properly in the art. As a result, you're losing a valuable training opportunity if you use your classroom time for non-Wing Chun related activities. If you do feel the need to do calisthenics, bodybuilding, or stamina training, you can (and should) do that outside of the Wing Chun classroom. In fact there are studies, which I strongly agree with, that prove that all a person needs to do to increase their fitness is 12 minutes of intense exercise in one session, once a week. For further information on this I would direct you to read the book *Body by Science* by Dr. Doug McGuff and John Little.

This is not to suggest that a good Wing Chun training program doesn't have health and fitness benefits. After all, we are using every aspect of our bodies—from multiple muscular contractions, to timing, to balance, to coordination, to breathing, and many more besides. As to the health and conditioning benefits of Wing Chun, I can attest that despite being in my sixties at the time of this writing, I routinely spar with students half my age and often twice my size, and yet I have no trouble overpowering them and can outlast them stamina-wise most of the time. One of my students was diagnosed with manic depression, and was on medication before starting Wing Chun. Now he's dropped his excess weight and medication. He's never felt better in his life.

There exists a very small percentage of women practicing Wing Chun these days. Most of them struggle in their classes. This is because the schools are running the wrong training program. They run a super macho program for men and women. They're trying to make men out of women instead of bringing out the femininity in both sexes. Recently, I trained a woman who had fifteen months of Wing Chun training in her country. She was really in bad shape as far as her Wing Chun performance was concerned. She had been taught to go as hard as possible with her fifty-seven-kilogram body and she was going nowhere with this approach. Lucky for her she had only invested two hours per week out of her fifteen months of training so that her bad habits were not too deeply ingrained. In three months I was able to turn her into a fighting machine by more fully cultivating the innate female nature in her. By contrast, her 6'3" and eighty-kilogram boyfriend, who had trained six to eight hours per week for those same fifteen months, struggled to make the change.

Macho men don't like to be associated with femininity; however, the truth of the matter is that men have female properties in them biologically. Men possess both an X and Y chromosome, whereas females have two X chromosomes. The Y chromosome is responsible, albeit not totally, for giving men their male characteristics, while the X chromosome is responsible for giving women their female characteristics. The spare X chromosome in men and women is generally inactive; however, it is not totally dormant; studies have shown that they are at least partially active. So, when I tell my male students to be more feminine, I'm really just telling them to activate this X chromosome that they already possess so that they can think and behave more like a female; i.e., less aggressively, less directly, and with more guile. They must follow the female path of fusion rather than the male pathology of domination.

Nowadays, Wing Chun is not taught, practiced, and represented as the founders had meant it to be. It is in a sad state today. I may sound like an elitist, but I would like to see Wing Chun go back to its original state of training where only the most serious, dedicated, and decent people were involved in it. Anything of any value loses its worth when it is diluted by the masses. It's time that Wing Chun was taught only to those who really deserve to be taught it.

I hope that the thoughts I am expressing will influence existing practitioners to make changes to both their attitude and training program, and will ensure that newcomers to Wing Chun start out on the right path. I have attempted to present a bigger, more complete picture of the jigsaw puzzle that is Wing Chun, but it is up to the individual practitioner to arrange these individual pieces of the puzzle on his own.

FOURTEEN

BUILDING AND PRESERVING STRENGTH

M ANY WING CHUN TEACHERS say that you must not use muscles but something inside called Qi (Chi). They also tell their students to relax, but do not specify *what* to relax.

Their instructions and belief regarding muscles are based on misinformation. After all, the reality is that if you don't use your muscles, nothing can move—you are essentially paralyzed. The Qi practitioners are forever searching for such a method of non-muscular movement, but they've never come close to obtaining it. There may be some who have found it in some form, but most of them are fakes or are in denial. I don't discount the existence of Qi, as I have practiced Qigong, and have felt it; however, I'm far from having the ability to use it effectively. So, for the time being, let's not discount muscles, and let's learn how to use them properly. As for relaxation, it is vital to understand what to relax. First off, you must learn to relax your mind—then you can learn how to relax the muscles that may oppose your action.

I have stated that in my Wing Chun classes, I do not focus on stamina or strength building through external conditioning exercises other than those outlined in the traditional Wing Chun curriculum as taught by Great-Grandmaster Ip Man. This is not to say that it is not necessary or beneficial to build (and particularly to retain) strength. I'm just saying that when you are in a Wing Chun class, I believe the focus should be on Wing Chun and that any other external conditioning you require should be done outside of the class. As it is, there just isn't enough time to work on Wing Chun alone to become proficient in it. So for the two or three hours that you are with me each session, I will focus just on Wing Chun.

As stated before, Wing Chun can take your existing potential to the maximum, whether you are a male, female, young, old, short, tall, thin, or fat. However, you can raise your potential by increasing your muscular strength as far as your body will allow. And while Wing Chun performance requires one to be soft, that is a matter of neural training and volition; i.e. one must choose to be soft and yet there is a yang element to the yin of softness and that is power (or force) production. And a stronger muscle is simply capable of producing more force than a weaker muscle and so it behooves the Wing Chun practitioner to keep his muscles as strong as possible for as long as he can. How much of the strength he chooses to employ in his Wing Chun training is entirely up to him (but it's nice to know that more is there for him when he needs it). A strength trainer such as my co-author, John Little, who specializes in this, has proven time and again that he can do this for you. In my many conversations with him I have learned exactly how and why you should train in a certain way to achieve the goals of enhanced strength, endurance, and health in the most economical, efficient, and productive way—strength training according to universal principles in much the same way that Wing Chun is human combat according to universal principles.

THE PROBLEM WITH (SOME) EXERCISE

We know that exercise is always (in as much as movement is involved) a source of wear and tear. We also know that exercise can bring punishing amounts of force to the body. And, to top it all off, it may or may not be good for you.

So why exercise at all? Simply because if we don't do *something* to preserve our muscular function the reality is that we will simply lose it, and, given that the life expectancy of our species is generally increasing, we don't want to spend the majority of our Autumn Years with decreased functional ability, nor do we wish to suffer from the various health problems that attend the progressive loss of muscle mass that afflicts the majority of the population who do not engage in some form of meaningful exercise. Many of our health problems stem from the loss (over time) of our Fast-Twitch muscle fibers—the ones that store the most glycogen, and thus, the ones that have a direct bearing on issues such as Type II Diabetes, high blood pressure, high cholesterol levels, and cardiovascular disease. The safest and most efficient manner to preserve and in some instances reclaim (and even enlarge) these fibers is through progressive resistance exercise.

And if you have detected an (at times not so subtle) attempt by the authors to suggest that resistance training might be a better way to go in your exercise pursuits, then you are absolutely correct. But this is not merely our opinion, despite being long-time advocates of resistance exercise. In a 2006 article in the *Canadian Medical Association Journal* that took as its thesis the review of all of the evidence regarding the benefits of exercise, the researchers concluded that resistance training represented a:

> paradigm shift...people with high levels of muscular strength have fewer functional limitations and lower incidences of chronic diseases such as diabetes, stroke, arthritis, coronary artery disease and pulmonary disorders...Musculoskeletal fitness is positively associated with functional independence, mobility, glucose homeostasis, bone health, psychological well-being, and overall quality of life, and is negatively associated with the risk of falls, illness, and premature death.[1]

THE CASE FOR RESISTANCE TRAINING

Resistance training leaps to the fore in terms of being the exercise of choice for the individual who has let go of such notions as "super health" and "miraculous transformations" and simply wants to achieve a better standard of fitness and muscular strength for him or herself that is not only safe but also sustainable. Resistance training engages one's muscles in a manner that involves as many metabolic pathways as possible, it requires the output of large amounts of energy when performed properly, and, at times, trips the growth and repair mechanism of the body into motion (we say "at times" as there is a genetic limit to one's ability to grow muscle), resulting in the individual trainee becoming stronger, leaner, and more capable of engaging in enjoyable activities that may not have been an option when the individual was weaker and less capable.

And while other forms of exercise can also accomplish this objective quite well,—running, cycling, swimming, gymnastics, rowing, and cross-country skiing come to mind—some of them (particularly in the case of running and cycling) only involve portions of the body and typically only the muscles and metabolic pathways of the lower extremities. In addition, all of these exercises bring a lot of wear and tear to the body and a rather weighty time investment. When the additional factor of safety is considered, resistance training emerges as, quite simply, the best option when choosing an exercise modality.

Quite apart from having a huge role in helping to shape one's appearance, strength training has produced a cavalcade of health benefits. In a blog posted on his website (www.bodybyscience.net), Emergency Room physician Doug McGuff, MD, indicated that proper resistance training delivered the following benefits to trainees:

1. It reverses age-related gene expression.
2. It increases Brain Derived Neurotrophic Factor (BDNF) elevations (an important mediator of improving brain functioning), which staves off or reverses age related cognitive decline and dementia.
3. It increases gut motility, which correlates with muscle mass. One's risk of gastro-intestinal cancer inversely correlates with gut motility.
4. It further plays a role in increasing internal organ mass (organ mass also correlates with muscle mass). If you should get in an accident or severely burn yourself, the time you have in the ICU before you die is correlated with organ mass. More muscle gives you more time on the clock.
5. If you were to get in a car accident, the kind of conditioning that strength training gives you may be the difference between three days of whiplash symptoms and a lifetime in a wheelchair (which will be a shortened lifetime).
6. High-intensity training enacts a hormonal cascade that is the antithesis of the metabolic syndrome, thus helping to stave off high blood pressure, elevated cholesterol levels, and obesity.
7. Enhances nitric oxide synthetase: you will have good blood pressure and will never need a little blue pill. You will not need to worry about "being healthy enough for sexual activity."
8. Bone mineral density correlates with muscle mass. Even in osteopenia, strong muscles absorb forces and prevent fractures.
9. Increases your Basal metabolism and hormonal profile, which helps to fight obesity.
10. You just look and feel good.

There is even some evidence that having more muscle and strength will help to stave off cancer.[2] So the "deal or no deal" question is: Would you be willing to tolerate no more than ten to twenty minutes of discomfort per workout along with a few minutes of post workout fatigue every seven to ten days if there was a chance that you could get stronger, move better, feel better, add some muscle and reduce your body fat? That would be a "deal" worth taking, particularly when compared to the other health and fitness "deals" that are being offered the general public that are long on hype but short on results.

We are of course aware that most people have their favorite exercise activity, but we would ask them to consider this: from cardiovascular fitness [3, 4] to muscular strength, to endurance, to flexibility, to the prevention of and rehabilitation from injury, to the relief of mental stress, resistance training can do it all, and it's the only method of exercise that involves all of these components of total fitness within a single method.

The health benefits associated with resistance training are considerable, including:

1. Decreased gastrointestinal transit time (reducing the risk of colon cancer) [5]
2. Increased resting metabolic rate [6]
3. Improved glucose metabolism [7]
4. Improved blood-lipid profiles [8, 9]
5. Reduced resting blood pressure [10, 11]
6. Improved bone mineral density [12]
7. Pain and discomfort reduction for those suffering from arthritis [13]
8. Decreased lower back pain [14, 15]
9. Enhanced flexibility [16]
10. Improved maximal aerobic capacity [17]

For those involved in Wing Chun or other martial arts, resistance training can stave off the potential for injury by strengthening joints, muscles, tendons, bones and ligaments, in addition to augmenting many of the attributes associated with physical performance, such as improving a practitioner's endurance, strength, power, speed, and vertical jump.[18] And, as we shall see, all of these benefits can be accomplished with a very minimal time investment.

While there are many protocols to choose from that require many different kinds of equipment, the fact that most people have (or can easily have) access to a basic barbell set will make this our preferred modality of exercise. Moreover, Danny Xuan's desire to go back to the intent and methods of the founders of Wing Chun has caused his co-author to reexamine the teachings of two of strength training's early pioneers. The method is a simple one—three sets of ten repetitions. And yet it may just be the most potent strength training protocol of all time. While we can split hairs (and often do) in strength training circles about such issues as free weights versus machines, slow reps versus faster reps, whether the gyms should be colder or warmer, whether you should do three exercises or five, or train once, twice or three times a week, for best results—none of the authorities in resistance training have produced anything close to the gains that have been produced by such a simple program of three sets of ten reps performed with a handful of multi-joint (or compound) exercises.

And three sets of ten, despite being dismissed by most as the most "basic" of strength and bodybuilding programs, nevertheless enjoys a track record of delivering very consistent results. Yes, there is context to consider; i.e., the fact that most of us had never been exposed to any form of strength training prior to our first workouts on the program that came with our first barbell set, and, thus, we were bound to respond well to it, however the fact remains that all of us *did respond well to it*; i.e., it *worked* (i.e., it built discernable muscle on our bodies). Moreover, this protocol (the exercises, the frequency, etc.) was not simply plucked out of thin air by every single barbell manufacturer to go along with their weight sets but rather was based upon the work of people who had studied resistance training and the effect it had on human muscle.

Given the quantity of mental calories we've been guilty of expending at such an extravagant rate on the subject of how best to exercise to increase our muscle size and strength over the decades, it's almost embarrassing to concede that few if any bodybuilding authors since the 1940s have put more muscle on more trainees with their programs than has the good ol' "three sets of ten" protocol that came with our first barbell set. Why?

THE WORK OF DELORME AND WATKINS

Because almost every strength training protocol that has been conceived over the past sixty years has been a footnote to the work of Thomas DeLorme and Arthur Watkins. DeLorme and Watkins were medical doctors who were perhaps the first to recognize the tremendous rehabilitation benefits afforded by resistance training during their work in helping wounded soldiers during World War II.

DeLorme was an orthopedic surgeon by profession but had lifted weights for many years prior to his professional work in rehabilitating soldiers. He knew from his own background as well as from his medical training that there was nothing about making an individual stronger that in any way posed a liability to that person's well-being. Indeed, he observed that making an individual stronger actually served as tremendous preventative medicine against that individual becoming infirm in the future. After achieving such remarkable success using resistance exercise in their rehabilitation of soldiers DeLorme and Watkins published the results of their work in

1951 in a book entitled *Progressive Resistance Exercise: Technic and Medical Application.* It became and remains the foundation of all variations of progressive resistance training.

The protocol that Delorme and Watkins found to be most successful was simple: three sets of ten repetitions for each exercise. The sequence moved from lighter to heavier weights with each successive set. This protocol, by means of more thoroughly warming up the targeted musculature, served to prevent injuries to muscles, tendons, ligaments, and joints. Moreover, the warm-up sets better prepared the muscles for the final and most demanding set (the "work set") to follow.[19]

I have found in training clients that it is important to get them accustomed to expending progressively higher amounts of energy (i.e., tapping the Fast-Twitch fibers that contain the most energy) and the DeLorme & Watkins method of performing three progressively heavier sets seems to ease the trainee into doing this quite nicely. The first set of ten repetitions can be considered a warm-up set that uses exclusively Slow-Twitch fibers; the second, a little heavier, set calls upon what's left of the Slow-Twitch fibers as well as bringing some Intermediate-Twitch Fibers into play; and the final, the heaviest, set fatigues out what's left of the Intermediate-Twitch fibers and brings the Fast-Twitch fibers into play, resulting in a protocol that maximizes fiber involvement and stimulates all of the metabolic processes of the body.

I have found that this protocol works best with three-to-five multi-joint or compound exercises, but more can be performed in a given workout using the same protocol if one's energy levels are particularly high or if one feels that one didn't quite give all that he or she had on the three-to-five exercises performed earlier.

Use a weight for each of these exercises that allows for ten repetitions. If your muscles start to fatigue after five or six repetitions to the point where seven repetitions is all you can do, the weight is too heavy. On the other hand, if you can do twenty or thirty repetitions, then the weight is obviously way too light. Make the adjustments and go to it, moving steadily from one exercise to the next. You should be able to complete your workout in less than twenty minutes.

No. 1: Military Press
Muscles: Upper back, Shoulders and Triceps.
Comment: This exercise works directly on the triceps and shoulders, but also strongly involves the clavicular portion of the chest, the abdominals and lower back. The triceps are underrated, but they play an important role in throwing and swimming, and they give balance to upper-arm strength.

Directions: Bend over, and using an overhand grip, hands about six inches apart, pick up the bar. Your feet should be about shoulder width apart. Stand up with your back straight, or sit straight on a bench. Bring the bar to a position directly over your head; then lower the bar slowly down to your upper chest. When the bar reaches your chest immediately change direction and press the bar back to the overhead position.

Reminder: Keep your back as straight as you can and your head up. This is not an easy exercise, so don't try to use too much weight at first.

No. 2: Bent-Over Rows

Muscles: Latissimus dorsi in the back, the trapezius in the neck, and the deltoids.

Comment: This exercise works the entire shoulder area, the smaller muscles of the back, and the broad latissimus muscles that span the back, the trapezius that supports the neck and shoulders, as well as the lower back and arms.

Directions: Stand with your feet comfortably spread. Keeping the legs as straight as possible (knees-locked position), bend over at the waist until your back is parallel with the floor. Take the bar in an overhand grip with the hands slightly wider than shoulder width, and bring the bar off the floor a few inches (if you have to bend the knees to pick up the bar, that's perfectly alright). Pull the bar to the chest without moving the upper body. Slowly lower the bar back to the starting position.

Reminder: This exercise is for the back primarily, but obviously the arms get some work as well. Don't let gravity take the bar away from the chest; keep the bar under control.

No. 3: Bench Press

Muscles: Pectorals, shoulders and triceps.

Comment: Since the chest, shoulders and triceps are all involved you'll be able to handle quite a bit of weight. It takes a certain amount of skill to raise and lower the weight in the proper form and under control so it may be helpful to practice with a light weight to get the feel of things. If you don't have a weight bench or a suitable substitute, you can do these presses on the floor or on an exercise mat.

Directions: Pick up the bar with an overhand grip, hands about shoulder width apart or a little wider. Bring the bar to your chest as you did for the squat (see No. 5, below), slowly sit down on the end of the bench, then lower yourself slowly until your back is flat on the bench and your head is resting comfortably. Keep your feet flat on the floor and slightly spread for leverage. Now press the bar straight up from the chest until your elbows are straight and your arms are fully extended. Pause at the top and lower the bar slowly and carefully until it just touches your chest. If you're using a bench, your elbows will be below the line of the bench in the bottom position. If you're on the floor, your elbows will touch the floor, and the bar may not quite touch your chest.

Reminder: Don't sit too close to the edge of the bench unless it is very stable because it might pop up behind you. Keep your buttocks on the bench at all times and try to arch your back slightly.

No. 4: Barbell Curls

Muscles: Biceps and Forearms.

Comment: The barbell curl is probably the simplest of the biceps exercises but it produces quick results. And it's still true that people tend to judge muscularity by the size of the biceps.

Directions: Bend over and pick up the bar with an underhand grip, hands a little more than shoulder width apart. Stand up and bring the bar up, using your legs and back until the bar is at arm's length in front of you—about mid-thigh. Keeping your feet comfortably spread, curl the bar up until it touches your chest. Make sure your back is straight and your head up throughout the exercise. Pause at the top and slowly lower the bar to the mid-thigh position.

Reminder: Try to keep your style and form during the curls. This means holding the shoulders back and using only the arms for leverage and the elbows as pivots. Lower the bar rather than letting it fall back to the starting position.

No. 5: Squats

Muscles: Upper legs, lower back, upper back.

Comment: Squats benefit the legs and the entire back as well, and they are good overall stimulators for the body because they involve most of the large muscles in one movement.

Directions: Stand with the feet comfortably spread. Make sure you have a strong, stable foundation. Bend over, flexing the knees, and grip the bar with an overhand grip, hands a little wider than shoulder width apart. Keep the head up and the back as flat as possible. Using the upper legs and lower back, bring the bar straight up in a plane parallel with the body. Keep the arms straight until the bar passes the knees, and then begin to bend the elbows and prepare to tuck them under the bar as it reaches chest level. Get underneath the bar and bring it to rest on the upper chest, just under the chin. Next, press the bar upward and then lower it behind your head so that it rests comfortably across the shoulders and the base of the neck. Adjust the weight and your stance until you're steady and well balanced, then squat as if sitting until your thighs are just below parallel. The feet should be flat on the floor at all times. Pause at the bottom to eliminate momentum that can be created by bouncing, and then slowly raise yourself back to the starting position.

Reminder: This is not an arm exercise. Use only the legs and back. Keep your head up at all times by focusing on the point where the ceiling meets the wall. If you're having any trouble with balance, try putting a small board under your heels.

OPTIONAL EXERCISES

No. 6: Stiff-Legged Deadlift
Muscles: Frontal thigh, hamstrings, buttocks, lower back.
Comment: The movements involved in the deadlift provide exercise for the lower back, strengthening the muscles and relieving tension at the same time. But this is really a good whole body exercise as well; it serves to prevent lower back problems, which are the most common medical complaints among athletes and the general public as well.
Directions: Take the same starting position as you did for the bent-over rows. Bend over at the waist, flexing the knees just a little, and grip the bar with an overhand/underhand grip, hands a little wider than shoulder width. Straighten the knees and lift the bar off the floor a few inches. Keep your back as flat as you can, and keep your head up. Now, keeping your knees straight, stand erect with the bar. Keep arms straight and shoulders back in the standing position. Bend over and lower the weight until it touches the floor.
Reminder: For the most benefit, be sure to exaggerate the shoulder movement when you reach the standing position by thrusting the shoulders back and the chest out. If you need to bend your knees more than suggested, go ahead and do so. You'll eventually be able to do the lift in proper form.

No. 7: Toe Raises
Muscles: Lower leg.
Comment: You can use a barbell placed across the top of your back (as in Squats) for this exercise, but we would recommend the use of dumbbells for both safety and balance reasons. This is the best and simplest exercise for strengthening the calf muscles.
Directions: Stand with your back straight, your head up, and the dumbbells held at your sides, palms in. If you're using a bar, let it hang down in

front of you with your arms fully extended. Lock your knees and rise up as high as you can on your toes. Hold at the top for a count of two and then slowly lower your heels back to the floor. If you want to increase the stretching motion, stand with your toes on a small block of wood, letting your heels touch the floor.

Reminder: Whether you use a block of wood or not, balance can be a problem with toe raises. With a little practice, however, you'll quickly get the hang of it.

No. 8: Bent-Leg Sit-Ups
Muscles: Abdominals.
Directions: Lie flat on your back on the floor and flex your knees until your feet also are flat on the floor. Hook your toes under a barbell, a bed, or anything that will hold them firmly. Put your hands behind your head. Next, curl your body up from the waist until your elbows touch your knees, and then lower yourself back to the starting position. Pause for a count of 2 and repeat. Start with 10 repetitions and add one sit-up every work-out. When you can do just about as many sit-ups as you want without get-ting sore stomach muscles, you can increase the intensity of the exercise by holding a light dumbbell behind your head.

Reminder: This is a stomach exercise, so if you feel any strain in your legs or back, increase your concentration and make sure the abdomen is getting the work. Don't bounce up from the floor because it will be momen-tum doing the work, not you.

As you can see, the exercises work the entire body, all the major muscle groups, and many of the minor ones as well—neck, upper back, shoulders, lower back, chest, biceps, triceps, buttocks, front thigh, hamstrings, calves, and abdomen. Four of the exercises work the legs; there are three for the back, three for the arms, two for the shoulders, and one each for the chest, buttocks and stomach. We suggest that you work out but once per week with this program as that is all that is required to both stimulate a strength increase and to allow your body the time it needs to produce a strength increase. Remember you are attempting to stimulate the growth and repair mechanism of the body into motion, much like a cut or burn will stimulate this mechanism into motion to produce new tissue to close a wound. And if you have ever noted how long it takes your body to produce the little bit of dermis or skin after the stimulus event of a burn or cut, it typically takes at least seven days. With strength training you are likewise tripping this growth and repair mechanism of the body into motion but this time you are looking to produce considerably more tissue than just enough to close a small wound. It stands to reason (and has been established empirically) that a seven-day interval is sufficient to allow your body to recover from the workout and to adapt by getting bigger and stronger. Training more frequently than is required is tantamount to burning yourself more frequently in an attempt to get your body to close a burn wound quicker.

This is just a baseline program, but a highly effective one. Every major muscle group is touched on with the first three exercises, and a little extra work is provided to muscles such as the biceps and triceps with exercises four and five. As you grow stronger, you may wish to experiment with dropping the direct arm exercises from time to time as a study published in *Applied Physiology, Nutrition, and Metabolism*[20] indicated that using an upper body pulling exercise (such as a Barbell Row or a Pulldown) worked just as well to stimulate the biceps muscles as did adding specific isolation exercises for the biceps to one's exercise program.

After several months, you may wish to reduce the frequency of your workouts even further, to once every 10 to 14 days as the bigger and stronger you get, the more fuel you're draining out of your "gas tank" (the muscles) and the longer it will take to refill them. If you prefer the once a week frequency, that's fine, but don't be worried about taking a few weeks off from strength training periodically, just to ensure that you are getting adequate recovery in between sessions to allow for optimal progress. We can't claim anything original in this program; it's simply a tried-and-true result-producing workout that can be performed with any barbell/dumbbell set. Other workout programs can make claims about being "more efficient," "stimulating greater growth," and being "state of the art," but these are, for the most part, simply marketing claims. The amount of muscle one can build is governed by certain biological and hormonal mediators, and most of us tap our potential for muscle mass within the first three years of training. What the "3 sets of 10" offers is a "bird in the hand," when it comes to *proven* muscle and strength building benefits. The other protocols, while perhaps effective, simply don't have the proven track record to be anything more (at this juncture anyway) than "two in the bush" (to follow through with our analogy).

EXERCISE PERFORMANCE

Now that we have an overview of the exercises and protocol, let's examine DeLorme's and Watkins's thoughts on how best to employ it. They advocated that each repetition one performs be initiated in a smooth and steady fashion, with no pause at the height of the movement or its termination at the initial starting position: "The load should be neither swung forward with a ballistic movement nor dropped under the influence of gravity."

In terms of repetitions, DeLorme and Watkins concede that, "the number of contractions per bout is arbitrarily set at ten." The reason they settled on ten is that, given the paucity of conclusive evidence on the matter (even to this day) combined with their empirical observations, that ten produced the desired results.

A frequent question from trainees is how long one should rest between sets of a given exercise. To this DeLorme and Watkins believed that one should rest only as long as is required in order for the trainee to be able to perform ten repetitions with the resistance once has chosen. They were quite clear in their writings, however, that prolonging the exercise or exercise session was a step in the wrong direction for the development of strength, writing:

> Whatever evidence exists tends to indicate that protracted exercise is not the prime requisite for the augmentation of strength. The power developed is important; that is, the amount of work done in unit time. Short-lived but intense exertion is the objective, which should be kept constantly in mind.

The first two of the three sets are, in effect, "warm up" sets; DeLorme and Watkins believed that the elevated temperature within the muscle had a positive effect on both the elastic and viscous components of muscle, which would assist the working muscles to perform their work due to "accelerating the chemical processes involved." In other words, by starting light and then working up in weight over three sets, the muscles being employed would be thoroughly warmed up by the time they were made to encounter the heaviest weight. Interestingly, they note that the warm up sets preceding the final set of ten repetitions actually allow for better performance on the final set: "Frequently patients are unable to perform ten repetitions with the 10-RM if this resistance is applied without preliminary exercise with lighter weights."

ONE SET IS ALL YOU REQUIRE

Interestingly, and very much in line with the authors' belief that only one all-out set is all that is necessary for optimal strength and size stimulation, DeLorme and Watkins concur. They stated [emphasis ours] that the benefits had

> *...by doing ten repetitions only with the 10-RM strength increases would be approximately the same as when three sets are performed.*

[211]

In fact, if it were not important to set the physiological stage preparatory to a maximum exertion, *only one set of ten repetitions would suffice. This has been demonstrated time and again in the clinic in the treatment of injuries in young athletes.*

So, if you're pressed for time or want to periodically change your protocol, simply take your working weight and perform one set to the point of muscular failure, or that point in a set where another repetition is no longer possible.

DeLorme and Watkins were also ahead of the curve with regard to intramuscular tension—rather than a certain number of repetitions—being an important factor in inducing hypertrophy: "Observations to date, though not conclusive, indicate that it is the tension the muscle is driven to develop that, to a great degree, if not entirely, is responsible for stimulating hypertrophy and consequently strength."

THE EFFECT OF RESISTANCE TRAINING ON MUSCLES

In terms of the effects on muscle size and endurance, the DeLorme and Watkins protocol is well documented by the authors, as they noted an increase in strength was accompanied by an increase in the measurable size of a muscle, which they attributed to the enlargement or hypertrophy of existing muscle fibers, as opposed to the creation of new fibers or hyperplasia. In addition, they noted an increase in the number of capillaries and the quantity of hemoglobin, glycogen and phosphocreatine, all of which resulted in a gain in muscular endurance in the trainee.

DeLorme and Watkins also cautioned against letting the total number of repetitions and sets get too high:

In the initial publications concerning progressive resistance exercise, seventy to one hundred repetitions were advocated, the repetitions being performed in seven to ten sets with ten repetitions per set. Further experience has shown that this figure is too high, and that in most cases a total of twenty to thirty repetitions is far more satisfactory. Fewer repetitions permit exercise with heavier muscle loads, thereby yielding greater and more rapid muscle hypertrophy.

In conclusion, then, the DeLorme and Watkins protocol has been time proven in its effectiveness. Rather than trying to reinvent the wheel or offer some new protocol that has yet to be tested for productivity, safety, and long-term compliance, it's always preferable to go with a sure thing—and three sets of ten is as close to that as has ever been offered in bodybuilding and strength training.

FIFTEEN

ON THE VALUE OF WING CHUN

ANTHROPOLOGISTS HAVE OFTEN WONDERED why America became the most developed, powerful and richest country in the world in just two centuries, while other countries with much longer histories and earlier civilizations have fallen back so far.

Some have answered by saying that the first immigrants had to find ways to fight and overcome the harshest winters, barren land, wild animals and the threat from other humans. Their will to survive and compete in all types of extremities made them strong, aggressive, determined, and inventive; whereas the people in the old countries became complacent from all the comforts that they had enjoyed for centuries.

I believe that Wing Chun was invented by women for the same reason; i.e., it was a matter of survival. Women have always been at a physical disadvantage when up against men. Traditionally, when villages were plundered by male marauders, the village men would be killed, and the women either raped or taken forcefully into the conquering culture. At some point the surviving women must have gotten together to devise a defense system for their villages. They may have lost many battles in the process, but eventually they learned how to maximize the potential of their smaller structure by using what we now know to be the laws of physics, which they may have learned from using simple farming and kitchen tools. Their fighting and defense system must have gotten stronger as time went by and eventually they were able to chase away the bandits. With the shortage of men in the village, they must have decided to create a matriarchal system, and vowed to keep it that way. The reputation of their strength must have traveled far and wide. Other villages must have eventually adopted the same or at least a similar system. Marauders began fearing these villages, and stopped attacking them.

There are anthropologists who believe that there was a time when there were more matriarchal villages than patriarchal, and that when the patriarchs finally were able to overpower the matriarchs they created a very suppressive environment for the matriarchs in order to ensure that they would never rise to power again.

I believe that the White Crane Temple was situated near one of these villages, and that Abbess Ng Mui visited it. She was inspired by the village women and used her martial arts experience to systematize her methods with theirs. Yim Wing Chun came to her in distress. Ng Mui took the opportunity to experiment and train Yim Wing Chun in the new system she had formulated. The system proved to be effective against the warlord who had pursued her. Later, Yim Wing Chun and her husband would go on to build upon this fighting concept, which was further developed by those who would become the inheritors of her art.

Historically, men have always developed martial arts; however, none of the arts created by men have ever been as simple yet complex, small yet full, delicate yet powerful, distinctive yet unclear, beautiful yet deadly as Wing Chun. Now, to my mind, that more perfectly describes the characteristics of a woman rather than a man.

Most martial arts that were created by males are based upon physical strength, stamina, and pain-tolerance conditioning. Some are based on the fighting movements of various animals, such as birds, insects, reptiles, tigers, and mythological creatures such as dragons. In contrast, Wing Chun's development was based on the human mind, the human body, and the human body's relationship with the Earth and the Universe; i.e., the laws that rule the universe. In this respect, Wing Chun can be considered the first "human"-inspired martial art, as it is based solely on our human attributes.

The human is the most developed, sophisticated, and intelligent animal in the world, so how would it make sense to try and ape (pardon the pun) a creature of lesser capacity? More specifically, we are not as strong as tigers, so why would we want to move in a manner that befits that animal's magnificent power and litheness when we fight? Moreover, we don't possess the tiger's long claws or sharp teeth, so what about how that animal fights has any relevance to our comparatively puny frames and sinews? But, again, we do possess a weapon that is greater than the greatest weapon of any other animal species—our brain. Therefore our fighting approach must be governed by this organ; it must make the best use of our greatest intellectual achievement; the understanding of the physical laws that govern our planet and our every movement. Our brains are unique in that they can receive, store and recall data. They have a super speed processor that can pick up data from storage and mutate it instantly to solve problems. Not only that, but our brains are even able to use existing data to create new data. Animals and insects simply do not possess this ability.

The major stumbling blocks on the path for men in their attempt to master Wing Chun are ego, masculine pride, and fear. These things get in the way of one's surrendering oneself wholeheartedly to the art. To fully embrace Wing Chun requires humility, femininity, and courage. Humility doesn't mean selflessness, but rather having confidence without aggrandizing oneself. Femininity doesn't mean emasculation, but knowing the female qualities that lie within each man and utilizing them. Courage doesn't mean fearlessness, but rather determination, dedication, and diligence.

Surrendering yourself to the art means trusting it enough to let it work for you. Most people are unable to let go of their ego, and enter into an art with preconceptions that they have picked up from movies, TV, or books and then work the art accordingly. What they need to do is discard their preconceptions and surrender to the art itself. However, the sad thing is that most teachers have the same misconceptions and therefore provide their students with exactly what they came looking for—a mindless, hard, and fast fighting product. The teacher demonstrates this by pounding the senior students, and the senior students demonstrate this by pounding the junior students, all the while feeding their own egos with pride and camouflaging the fears they have within. They do that at any cost, veering away from the keys that will unlock the highest levels of the very art to which they've dedicated themselves.

Many movies have presented Wing Chun as a hard and fast fighting system for macho men who eliminate dozens of opponents with lightning fast hands and feet. Such a presentation attracts people with inner fears who want to overcome them. Whenever such movies come out there is always a surge in enrollment in Wing Chun schools. However, the true concept and art of Wing Chun remains hidden to such filmmakers and, by extension, their audiences.

Wing Chun is both an art and a culture. Art is something beautiful and expressive. Culture is something traditional and characteristic of a people. That is all being destroyed and bastardized by those who have no respect and appreciation for the art and culture. Wing Chun is a Chinese fighting concept and culture. It is an art that was developed originally by women who later passed it on to men who were able to maintain the feminine approach and yet adapt it to the male structure.

[217]

The concept underpinning Wing Chun is to treat yourself as always having a physical disadvantage, which will cause you to rely on skill rather than force. Skills are acquired by understanding the laws of physics and biomechanics, and by developing your body and mind so that they work together to your advantage. The laws of physics and biomechanics are a study of force. When you understand the nature of force, you can use this knowledge in any circumstance and within any environment and against any kind of force or opponent.

It must be noted that most of the greats of martial arts were men of small stature such as Ip Man of Wing Chun, Yang Luchan of Yang Tai Chi, Dong Haichuan of Baguazhang, Jigoro Kano of Judo, Morihei Ueshiba of Aikido, and Gichin Funakoshi of Karate. They averaged 5'3" (160 centimeters). They didn't have assertive statures, but found a way to make themselves assertive through their arts.

In order to instill the Wing Chun concept of fighting, a special training is required. The training involves application of the knowledge of structures, so that one knows how to align one's body in a manner that will produce the most economical, efficient and productive use of one's energy in the art of combat. Thus, the arm and body positions in Wing Chun, along with movements such as the Tansau, Bongsau, Fooksau, Gangsuo, Sun punch and rear-weighed horse were developed for this purpose.

Once you have been armed with the best shields and weaponry, Wing Chun training provides you with fighting strategies, one of which is to always have visual and physical contact with your opponent so that you can readily discern his strengths, weaknesses, and movements. This strategy calls for you to not simply charge blindly into an incoming force, but to evaluate it first before deciding on the best course to take—be it to yield, deflect, dissipate, or counterattack it. Because of your physical disadvantage you must use your larger bones and muscles against your opponent's smaller ones; you must lash out with all three limbs simultaneously against one of his; you must strike at the opponent's vital points where he has no muscular protection. Every defense must include offense, and every offense must include defense. All of these strategies will work best when you are constantly in touch with your opponent.

One of Confucius' teachings is to humble yourself and to put others above you; to always be kind, polite, and helpful. So, if you invite someone over for dinner, you don't wait for him to come to your house but go to meet him at his house and bring him into your home. When he leaves you don't just wave goodbye from your door but accompany him back to his house. When you have invited someone to your home, these are your obligations and preoccupations. When you don't engage yourself in any appointment, you are free from obligation, thus, free to go anywhere you wish.

From this cultural perspective came the saying in Wing Chun, "Receive him when he comes; go with him when he leaves; and go freely when there is no engagement." In Wing Chun's interpretation, it means make contact to receive the opponent's incoming force and dissipate it; maintain contact with it and follow the opponent's retreat with an attack; and if there is no engagement, then attack your opponent freely.

This philosophy is completely in accord with Sun Tzu's strategy on warfare; that is, to know your enemy and yourself, and to use deceit, surprise and indirect attacks to win the war.

One thing that Sun Tzu was adamant about was that it is better to win opponents over than it is to conquer them. The reason being that the cost in terms of manpower, money, and time in waging war far outweighs the cost of the same via peaceful negotiation. In terms of Wing Chun training you must know how to win a fight without fighting. This is the epitome of accomplishing a task with minimum economy, maximum efficiency, and productivity. You must learn to negotiate with your opponent and, if necessary, swallow your pride and lose a smaller battle in order to win a bigger war. After all, winning some battles may only set you up to have to engage in a protracted and draining war that lasts far too long and takes too great a toll on you. And these are hard lessons to abide when one has a large amount of pride and ego.

If one doesn't recognize these elements of Chinese culture in Wing Chun, it will prove exceedingly difficult to incorporate these philosophies into your education and understanding of the art. As indicated earlier, the ones who do not understand the deeper aspects of the art can be readily seen on YouTube these days; the epitome of "all flash and no substance."

Wing Chun was designed for self-protection in the strictest sense. In this respect it can be likened to wearing the seatbelt in your car. You may never get into an accident, but if you ever do that seatbelt will provide you with a far greater chance of surviving the accident than if you didn't have it on. With that insurance you can enjoy your driving and smell the roses, too. Similarly, you may never get into a fight but, if you do, your Wing Chun training can provide you with a much better chance of emerging from it unscathed or with minimal damage from such an encounter (or even getting out of it alive). Even if you never have to use Wing Chun the time and effort you invest into your training will have been worth it as you will be rewarded with good health, a better understanding of Chinese culture and art, and, most of all, you will be equipped with nature's greatest tools to help you deal successfully with all of the conflicts of human existence.

GLOSSARY OF CHINESE CHARACTERS AND TERMS

Chinese Trad/ Sim	Romanized Cantonese	Cantonese Variables	Romanized Mandarin (Pronounce)	Meaning
詠	Wing	Ving	Yong (Yoong)	Poem, Song, Recital
永	Wing	Wing, Wen	Yong	Forever, Always, Perpetual, Everlasting
春	Chun	Tsun	Chun (Troon)	Spring Season/Time
拳	Kuen	Kyun	Quan (Chuan)	Fist, Punch, Boxing, Pugilism
法	Fat	Faat	Fa	Method, Methodology, Law, Management
葉, 叶	Ip	Yip	Yie	Leaf, Page
問, 问	Man	Man	Wen	Question, Inquisitive
小	Siu	Seu	Xiao (Sheow)	Small, Little, Fundamentals, Basic
念	Nim	Lim	Nian	Read, Study, Idea, Thought
頭, 头	Tau	Tao, Tou, To	Tou (Thow)	Head, Top, Beginning, First, Main
尋, 寻	Chum	Cham	Xun (Shuin)	Seek, Search, Hunt

Chinese Trad/ Sim	Romanized Cantonese	Cantonese Variables	Romanized Mandarin (Pronounce)	Meaning
橋, 桥	Kiu	Ku	Qiao (Chiow)	Bridge, Connection
鏢, 镖	Biu	Bu	Biao (Pbiow)	Hurl, Dart, Throw
指	Jee	Ji, Zi	Zhi (Treuh)	Finger, To Point,
木	Muk	Mook	Mu (Moo)	Wood, Wooden
人	Yan	Yun, Yen, Jan	Ren	Man, Person, People
椿, 桩	Jeong	Jong, Zong	Zhuang (Truaang)	Stump, Stake, Post
六	Luk	Look, Lok	Liu (Leeow)	Six
點, 点	Dim	Din	Dian (Tdien)	Point, Dot, O'Clock
半	Boon	Bun, Poon	Ban (Pbaan)	Half, Incomplete
桿, 杆	Gon	Gwan, Kwan, Kun, Koon	Gan (Kgaan)	Pole, Staff, Stick
八	Bat	Baat	Ba (Pbaa)	Eight, Shape
斬, 斩	Jum	Jam, Cham, Chaam, Zaam	Zhan (Traan)	Cut, Cut Off, Hack, Slice, Behead
刀	Do	Dou	Dao (Tdaow)	Knife, Single-Edged Sword, Blade
館, 馆	Gun	Gwon, Kwon, Koon, Kun	Guan (Kguen)	Establishment, Premises, School, Gym, Building, Shop
手	Sau	Sao	Shou (Rsheow)	Hand, Arm, Hand and Arm Position, Shape or Action, Hand Skills
脚	Gerk	Geuk	Jiao (Chjiow)	Foot, Leg, Foot and Leg Position, Shape or Action
攤, 摊	Tan	Taan	Tan (Thaan)	Spread Out, Spread Open, Extend, Expand
伏	Fook	Fuk	Fu	Prostrate, Lie Low, Conceal, Submit, Subdue, Cover, Ambush

Chinese Trad/ Sim	Romanized Cantonese	Cantonese Variables	Romanized Mandarin (Pronounce)	Meaning
膀	Bong	Pong	Bang (Pbaang)	Wing, Wing Action, Upper Arm
護, 护	Wu	Woo	Hu (Hoo)	Guard, Protect, Defend, Safeguard
欄, 拦	Lan	Laan	Lan	Bar, Rail, Barrier
問, 问	Man	Mun	Wen (Wun)	Probe, Inquest
圈	Huen	Hyun	Quan (Choo'ean)	Circle, Loop
窒	Jad	Jat, Zat	Zhi (Treuh)	Stop, Obstruct, Brake, Stifle, Dampen
拍	Pak	Paak	Pai (Pie)	Clap, Pat
臘, 拉	Lap	Lab, Lat	La	Pull, Drag, Seize
打	Da	Ta, Taa, Daa	Da (Tdaa)	Strike, Hit, Punch, Fight, Shoot
踢	Tek	Tik	Ti (Thee)	Kick
跆	Toi	Toy	Tai (Thai)	Kick, Trample
滾	Gwan	Guan, Kwan	Gun (Kgoon)	Roll, Roll Away, Roll Out, Stir, Boil, Get Rid Of
耕	Gang	Gan, Kang	Geng (Kgeng)	Plow, Till, Dig
跟	Gan	Kan	Gen (Kgen)	Heel, Follow Closely
掌	Jeong	Jong, Chong	Zhang (Trang)	Palm, Open-Palm
正	Jing	Zing, Jin, Ching	Zheng (Treng)	Upright, Straight
二	Yi	Yee	Er	Two
字	Ji	Jee	Zi (Tzeuh)	Chinese Character, Letter, Word, Symbol
箝	Kim	Gim	Qian (Chi'ean)	Clamp
羊	Yeung	Yung, Joeng	Yang	Sheep, Lamb
馬, 马	Ma	Maa	Ma	Horse, Lower Trunk (in Martial Arts)
身	Seong	San	Shen (Rshen)	Body, Structure

Chinese Trad/Sim	Romanized Cantonese	Cantonese Variables	Romanized Mandarin (Pronounce)	Meaning
偏	Pian	Pin	Pian (Pi'ean)	Slant, Oblique, Angled
道	Dao	Tao, Dou, Do	Dao (Tdaow)	The Way, Method, Path, Principle, Reason
套	Tao	Tou	Tao (Thao)	Form, Pattern, Sequence, Standard, Set
路	Lu	Lou, Lo	Lu (Loo)	Road, Journey, Path, Way
型	Jing	Kata (Japanese)	Xing (Shing)	Pattern, Form, Template
訣	Kuit	Kyut	Jue (Chjue)	Secret, Secret of an Art
黐	Chi	Ci, Tse	Chi (Triue)	Sticky, Sticking, Stickiness
意	Ji	Jee, Chi	Yi	Intent, Intention, Idea, Thought,
力	Lik	Leek	Li	Strength, Power, Force
中	Cheong	Zung, Chong	Zhong (Troong)	Center, Central, Middle, Core
心	Sam	Sim	Xin (Shin)	Heart, Mind, Soul, Core
線, 线	Sin	Seong	Xian (She'ean)	Line, Route, Path, Plane, Thread, Track, Chord
忠	Zung	Tsung, Chung	Zhong (Troong)	Devoted, Honest, Loyal
衷	Cheong	Cung, Zung	Zhong (Troong)	Inner Feelings, Emotion, Intention
功	Kung	Gung	Gong (Kgoong)	Skill, Art, Effort, Hard Work, Training
內	Noi	Noy	Nei	Internal, Inner, Inside
夫	Fu	Fu	Fu (Foo)	Man, Laborer
氣, 气	Hei	Hey	Qi (Chee)	Air, Vital Energy, Properties of Air
單, 单	Dan	Daan	Dan (Dtaan)	Single, Solo, Odd Number
雙, 双	Soeng	Sueng	Shuang (Rshuang)	Double, Pair, Dual
唐	Tong	Kara (in Japanese)	Tang (Thang)	Tang Dynasty (618-907); Chinese People of that Era

Chinese Trad/ Sim	Romanized Cantonese	Cantonese Variables	Romanized Mandarin (Pronounce)	Meaning
空	Hung	Kara (in Japanese)	Kong (Khoong)	Empty, Emptiness, Unoccupied, Space
日	Jat	Jut	Ri (Re'ue)	Sun, Day, Date
Compound Words				
詠春拳法	Wing Chun Kuen Fat		Yong Chun Quan Fa	Methodology of the "Springtime Recital" Fists
小念頭	Siu Nim Tau		Xiao Nian Tou	Fundamental Studies in the Beginning; Small Idea in the Head
尋橋	Chum Kiu		Xun Qiao	Seeking the Bridge; Seeking Connection
鏢指	Biu Jee		Biao Zhi	Hurling the Fingers
木人桩	Muk Yan Jong		Mu Ren Zhuang	Wooden Man Post
六點半桿	Luk Dim Boon Goon		Liu Dian Ban Gan	Six and a Half Staff
八斬刀	Bat Jum Dou		Ba Zhan Dao	Eight Cutting Sword Form
黐手	Chisau		Chi Shou	Sticking Arms, Connecting Arms
黐脚	Chigerk		Chi Jiao	Sticking Legs
二字箝羊馬	Yi Ji Kim Yeung Ma		Er Zi Qian (Chi'ean) Yang Ma	Character Two Clamping Goat Horse (Stance)
日字拳	Jat Yi Kuen		Ri Zi Quan	Sun Character Fist
攤打	Tan Da		Tan Da	Extend Open Palm Hand and Strike Simultaneously
拉大	Lap Da		La Da	Pull Opponent's Arm and Strike Simultaneously
拍打	Pak Da		Pai Da	Pat the Opponent's Arm and Strike Simultaneously
中心	Cheong Sam		Zhong Xin	Core, Center Core

Chinese Trad/ Sim	Romanized Cantonese	Cantonese Variables	Romanized Mandarin (Pronounce)	Meaning
中心線	Cheong Sam Sin		Zhong Xin Xian	Center Core Line
中线	Cheong Sin		Zhong Xian	Centerline Plane, Centerline Path
衷心	Cheong Sam		Zhong Xin	Ernest (from the heart)
忠心	Cheong Sam		Zhong Xin	Devotion (from the heart)
正掌	Jing Jeong		Zhen Zhang	Upright Palm
偏掌	Pian Jeong		Pian Zhang	Slant Palm
正身馬	Jing Seong Ma		Zheng Shen Ma	Front-Body Horse, Front-Facing Horse
偏身馬	Pian Seong Ma		Pian Shen Ma	Slant-Body Horse, Side-Facing Horse
氣功	Hei Gung		Qigong	Revitalizing Exercise
功夫	Kung Fu		Gong Fu	Labored Skill, Skill Acquired from Hard Work or Training, Manpower
內功	Noi Kung		Nei Gong	Internal Power, Internal Work, Internal Skills
唐手	Tongsau	Karate (Japanese)	Tang Shou	The Way of the Chinese Hands
空手	Hungsau	Karate (Japanese)	Kung Shou	The Way of the Empty Hands
前頂	Cin Deng		Qian Ding	Front Crown (In Chinese Medicine, it is the Meridian located at the apex of the head)
會陰	Wui Jam		Huiyin	Returning to Shade (In Chinese Medicine, it is located at the middle of the perineum)
佛山	Fatsan		Foshan	Buddhist Mountain (Ip Man's Birthplace)
葉問	Ip Man		Yie Wen	Inquest Page, Inquisitive Leaf

Notes on the Text

PREFACE

1. Source: Laotse, *The Book of Tao*, LXXVIII. Lin Yutang translation, pages 622–623, *The Wisdom of China and India*, Random House, © 1942.)

CHAPTER FOURTEEN

1. Warburton, Darren, Crystal Whitney Nicol, and Shanon Bredin. "Health Benefits of Physical Activity: The Evidence." Canadian Medical Association Journal 174 (2006): 801-9.

2. Researchers studied patients with advanced melanoma to understand the illness as it related to muscle strength. They looked at CT scans of the psoas muscle in order to measure core muscle density. The authors then correlated the core muscle density with the risk of metastasis, or spreading of the cancer. Patients with higher muscle density were found to have significantly better survival rates and less metastasis. The authors concluded that decreased muscle density was an important predictor in the outcome of the disease. Furthermore, they stated that, "frailty, not age, was associated with decreased disease-free survival."

Here is the abstract: Sarcopenia as a Prognostic Factor among Patients with Stage III Melanoma

Background: Several hypotheses proposed to explain the worse prognosis for older melanoma patients include different tumor biology and diminished host response. If the latter were true, then biologic frailty, and not age, should be an independent prognostic factor in melanoma.

Methods: Our prospective institutional review board (IRB)-approved database was queried for stage III patients with computed tomography (CT) scans at time of lymph node dissection (LND). Psoas area (PA) and density (PD) were determined in semi-automated fashion. Kaplan-Meier (K-M) survival estimates and Cox proportional-hazard models were used to determine PA and PD impact on survival and surgical complications.

Results: Among 101 stage III patients, PD was significantly associated with both disease-free survival (DFS) (P = 0.04) and distant disease-free survival (DDFS) (P = 0.0002). Cox multivariate modeling incorporating thickness, age, ulceration, and N stage showed highly significant association with PD and both DFS and DDFS. DDFS was significantly associated with Breslow thickness (P = 0.04), number of positive nodes (P = 0.001), ulceration (P = 0.04), and decreasing muscle density (P = 0.01), with hazard ratio of 0.55 [95% confidence interval (CI) 0.35-0.87]. PD also correlated with surgical complications, with odds ratio (OR) of 1.081 [95% CI 1.016-1.150, P = 0.01].

Conclusions: Decreased psoas muscle density on CT, an objective measure of frailty, was as important a predictor of outcome as tumor factors in a cohort of stage III melanoma patients. On multivariate analysis, frailty, not age, was associated with decreased disease-free survival and distant disease-free survival, and higher rate of surgical complications.

3. Steele, J; Fisher, J; McGuff, D.; Bruce-Low. S; Smith, D. Resistance Training to Momentary Muscular Failure Improves Cardiovascular Fitness in Humans: A Review of Acute Physiological Responses and Chronic Physiological Adaptations. Journal of Exercise Physiology On-Line, Volume 15 Number 3 June 2012; 53-80.

4. Messier, S.P., Dill, M.E. Alterations in strength and maximum oxygen consumption consequent to nautilus circuit weight training. *Res Q Exerc Sport* 1985; 56: 345-51.

5. Koffler, K., Menkes, A., Redmond, A., et al. Strength training accelerates gastrointestinal transit in middle-aged and older men. *Med Sci Sports Exerc* 1992; 24: 415-9.

6. Campbell W, Crim M, Young C, et al. Increased energy requirements and changes in body composition with resistance training in older adults. *Am J Clin Nutr* 1994; 60: 167-75.

7. Hurley B. Does strength training improve health status? *Strength Cond J* 1994; 16: 7-13.

8. Stone M, Blessing D, Byrd, R., et al. Physiological effects of a short-term resistive training program on middle-aged untrained men. *Nat Strength Cond Assoc J* 1982; 4: 16-20.

9. Hurley B, Hagberg, J., Goldberg A., et al. Resistance training can reduce coronary risk factors without altering VO2 max or percent body fat. *Med Sci Sports Exerc* 1988; 20: 150-4.

10. Harris K.A., Holly R.G. Physiological responses to circuit weight training in borderline hypertensive subjects. *Med Sci Sports Exerc* 1987; 19: 246-52.

11. Colliander E..B, Tesch, P.A. Blood pressure in resistance trained athletes. *Can J Appl Sport Sci* 1988; 13: 31-4.

12. Menkes A., Mazel S., Redmond A., et al. Strength training increases regional bone mineral density and bone remodeling in middle-aged and older Men. *J Appl Physiol* 1993; 74: 2478-84

13. Rall, L.C., Meydani S.N., Kehayias, J.J., et al. The effect of progressive resistance training in rheumatoid arthritis: increased strength without changes in energy balance or body composition. *Arthritis Rheum* 1996; 39: 415-26.

14. Nelson, B.W., O'Reilly E., Miller, M., et al. The clinical effects of intensive specific exercise on chronic low back pain: A controlled study of 895 consecutive patients with 1-year follow up. *Orthopedics* 1995; 18: 971-81.

15. Risch, S., Nowell, N., Pollock, M., et al. Lumbar strengthening in chronic low back pain patients. *Spine* 1993; 18: 232-8.

16. Westcott W. Keeping Fit. *Nautilus* 1995; 4: 50-7.

17. Messier, S.P., Dill, M.E. Alterations in strength and maximum oxygen consumption consequent to nautilus circuit weight training. *Res Q Exerc Sport* 1985; 56: 345-51.

18. Stone, MH. Muscle conditioning and muscle injuries. *Med Sci Sports Exerc* 1990; 22: 457-62.

19. According to Shellock and Prentice (1985) most of the physiological effects of warm up are temperature dependent. Muscle contraction requires the breaking of adenosine tri-phosphate (ATP) to provide the energy for cross-bridge formation (see Sliding Filament Mechanism, Norkin and Levangie, 2000, p277). According to Marieb (1998) only 20–25% of the energy produced through muscle contraction goes towards directly functional work. The remaining 75-80% is given off as heat. It is this heat that causes the rise in tissue temperature that is so advantageous to the athlete.

The physiological effects of raised muscle temperature are numerous. Increased body temperature increases oxygen delivery to the working tissues by facilitating oxygen dissociation from hemoglobin and myoglobin (Shellock and Prentice, 1985).

Vasodilation occurs as a result of increased temperature and waste production (Karvonen, 1978). Local vasodilation redistributes blood from the viscera to working muscles. This shunting of blood flow allows increased nutrient and oxygen delivery and improves the efficiency of waste product removal.

20. Gentil, Paulo, Sampaio Soares, Rodrigo, Pereira, Maria Claudia, Rodrigues da Chunha, Rafael, Martorelli, Saulo Santos, Martorelli, Andre Santos, Bottaro, Martim, Effect of adding single-joint exercises to a multi-joint exercise resistance-training program on strength and hypertrophy in untrained subjects. Applied Physiology, Nutrition, and Metabolism, 2013, 38 (3): 341-344, 10.1139/apnm-2012-0176.

AUTHORS' NOTES

1. Biotensegrity: After studying and practicing martial arts for over fifty years, I can consider myself somewhat of an expert—at least in Wing Chun. To understand how the human body and mind works, I read every material I can get hold of regarding human anatomy, neurology, kinesiology, biomechanics, physics, and human architecture, design, and science. However, I'm by no means an expert in these fields. I came upon the subject of Tensegrity and Biotensegrity about ten years ago, and was fascinated by them. I shared the information on my website to those who had subscribed to it, and now share it in this book. For fear of misinterpreting such a complex subject I contacted Dr. Stephen M. Levin MD, the very person who coined the term Biotensegrity, requesting permission to use some of his writings. With his approval, I have taken excerpts from his various articles and inserted them in the Biotensegrity, The Sacrum, and Triangulation sections found in Chapter Ten. I thank him kindly for his generosity. For those interested in knowing more about Biotensegrity, go to Dr. Stephen Levin's website, www. biotensegrity.com.

2. Transliteration of the Chinese Language: Like many other languages, the Chinese language has sounds that are unique to it, and not available in the English language. To compound the problem, the Chinese have multiple colloquial languages and dialects. Historically, China didn't become a united country until the end of 221 B.C.E under the Qin Dynasty. Prior to that, it was made up of many independent kingdoms, with each having its own language, culture, and standards—such as monies and measures. After conquering and unifying the "Warring States" the first emperor of China, Qin Shi Huangdi (秦始皇帝) degreed a single language and standardization of

measurements. After studying and selecting the most practical and efficient language (in his opinion) from works submitted by scholars from the old kingdoms, he burnt their books and executed the uncooperative scholars. Although he was able to standardize the written language, he was unable to standardize the spoken language. So, although 吃 would represent *eat*, one region of people will say *Chi*, and another region will say *Sik*, because that's how they had always said *eat* it in their languages.

In China, there are fifty-six different ethnic groups recognized officially by the government. They are differentiated by their uniqueness in language, food, culture, and attire. The largest majority are the Han Chinese, which populate most of China. The rest of the other ethnic groups reside mostly in Western China; particularly in the Yunnan province. In Western China, the ethnic groups speak entirely different languages; however, the schools all teach them the official Chinese language called Guoyu (國語—National Language) or Putonghua (普通話—Common Dialect) or Zhongwen (中文—Chinese/Central Literary) or Hanyu (漢語—Han People's Language) or Mandarin—as coined by the early Westerners visiting China who noted the language spoken by the Chinese court bureaucrats whom they also called Mandarins.

The first Westerner to publish a transliteration or Romanization of the "Mandarin" language was British Ambassador, Thomas Wade in 1867; it was later revised by another British diplomat Herbert Giles and his son Lionel, in 1912; the system came to be known as Wade-Giles. Although it was widely used in the English-speaking world, it wasn't always used in China, Asia, or other Western countries because of how the Roman alphabets were pronounced there. Also, the Wade-Giles system was confusing and inconsistent, making it difficult to understand unless someone spent a lot of time studying the system. The system wasn't entirely to be blamed because the Roman alphabets just didn't have equivalent sounds to some Chinese sounds. For example, there is no exact equivalent to the English *b* sound in Chinese; however, there is a sound that is a cross between *b* and *p*. There is a *p* sound though, and is pronounced like in English, with an *h* aspiration; i.e., *pink* pronounced as *phink*. The Chinese *p-b* cross sound is pronounced *p* without the *h* aspiration, i.e. pronouncing *pink* without the *h* aspiration. To separate the two, Wade-Giles allocated *p* for the non-aspirated sound, and allocated p with an apostrophe *p'* for the aspirated sound. That was done for other sounds like t and k, which in Chinese have aspirated and non-aspirated sounds. For example, k represented the non-aspirated sound, and k' represented the aspirated sound. So, Kung Fu was supposed to be pronounced without aspiration; whereas, K'ung Fu would be pronounced

Khung Fu, which is how Westerners pronounce Kung Fu. In fact K'ung Fu (Khung Fu) could end up meaning Empty Skills, which is quite the opposite of Kung Fu, meaning Highly Skilled. To make matters worse, Wade-Giles allocated another sound to the k for some unknown reason. It was to sound like a cross between *j* and *ch*. Here again, there is no equivalent sound of *j* in Chinese; however, there are two sounds for *ch*; i.e., one with aspiration and one without. In English, the word chicken is pronounced with aspiration. Imagine pronouncing without aspiration; that is what Wade-Giles allocated the k sound for it as well. So, for the capital of China, 北京, they transliterated as Peking, which is supposed to be read as Pe (*P* without aspiration, and e pronounced as *uh*), ching (*ch* without aspiration). As we know now, it was never pronounced that way, but the way it appears. Although Wade and Giles were British diplomats, I'm unaware if they were linguists. That may have been the problem. To be proficient in a language, the requirement isn't just knowing how to sound out the words, but having excellent hearing for sounds. With China having so many dialects—some estimating as many as eight thousand, Wade and Giles may not have worked with the right people or didn't have the ears for languages, thus may have heard the words wrong and transliterated them wrong. On the other hand, there are dialects in China that pronounce China's capital as Pak King ... but certainly not by the Mandarins of the court. So, perhaps Wade and Giles heard it that way and transliterate that way—Peking.

In 1958, the Chinese government systemized and implemented its own transliteration system called Pinyin (拼音). It is not without complications, but only because of the language's unfamiliar sounds and tones. It is by far superior, simpler, and more accurate than Wade-Giles system. For example, *b* was allocated for the non-aspirated *p* sound, and *p* was left to sound aspirated as English speakers would say it. Instead of using *k* as Wade-Giles did for the non-aspirated *ch* sound, it allocated *j*. Thus the Capital was transliterated as Beijing instead of Peking. Although people who do not understand the Pinyin system still pronounce Beijing incorrectly and as it appears, it is by far closer to the actual sound than Peking. The correct way of pronouncing it would be Pei (without the aspiration) Ching (without the aspiration).

In Pinyin, 功夫, is transliterated as Gongfu instead of Kung Fu, thus pronounced Koong (without aspiration) Foo. 太极 is transliterated as Taiji, and pronounced Thai (with aspiration) Chee (without aspiration) instead of Tai Chi. 氣功 is transliterated as Qigong, and pronounced Chee (with aspiration) Koong (without aspiration), instead of Chi Kung. Although the Q can throw a reader off, one just has to learn to allocate the Chee (with aspiration) sound to it. It is no different than pronouncing *J* as *H* in another language.

Although Wade-Giles allocated Ch' (with the apostrophe) for the non-aspirated sound, writers ignored it and simple wrote it without the apostrophe. Consequently, those with no knowledge of the Chinese language often think of Chi used in both Tai Chi and Chi Kung being the same. However, when you examine the Chinese characters for them, 极 and 氣, they are entirely different in appearance, sound, and meaning. 极 is pronounced Chee without aspiration and written as *ji* in Pinyin, means ultimate; therefore, 太 极— Taiji would mean The Greatest Ultimatum. Whereas, 氣—Chi in Chi Kung, written as Qi in Pinyin, means Air or Properties of Air; therefore, 氣 功 would mean the Study of Air and its Properties.

In this book, I've mainly used the Pinyin transliterations; however, the publisher felt that certain words should be left the way English speakers are familiar with, such as Tai Chi, Kung Fu, and Tao. In fact, I had initially used Dao instead of Tao for the title and inside the book. Here again, in the Chinese language, there are two *t* sounds; one with aspiration, and one without. In English, when you say *two*, you actually pronounce it *thoo*. In Chinese, there is a *t* sound without the *h* aspiration. It sounds more like how some Europeans say *two*. Pinyin allocated *d* for this sound. So, when you talk about the Chinese philosophy, The Way, it should be written as Daoism or the Dao—道. Whereas, when you refer to the forms or shadow-boxing patterns in a martial arts system, it should be written as Tao—套. However, for marketing purposes, the title was changed to The Tao of Wing Chun for easy recognition.

In 1958, the Chinese Government not only transliterated the Chinese language, it also changed the written script. It simplified it by removing strokes from words that had many. It was referred as Simplified Chinese. Although the billion Chinese in Mainland used this script, overseas Chinese continued using the old script. To differentiate the two, the old script was referred as Traditional Chinese. It is used by the Chinese in Hong Kong, Taiwan, Southeast Asia, Americas, and Europe. Because Wing Chun is associated with Hong Kong, particularly from Ip Man's lineage, I have chosen to use the Traditional script wherever I use Chinese.

The Chinese government only officially transliterated the National Language, Mandarin, as it is known in the West. It did not transliterate the other languages or dialects. Although there are transliterations by Yale University, Hong Kong Government, and others for the Cantonese tongue, none are considered official or a standard; thus, you will see Chow, Chao, or Chou for the same surname 周, or Law, Low, Lowe, Lau, Liu, Lui, Louie for another popular surname 劉. Even within Canton or Guangdong province, there are many different Cantonese dialects. Consequently, we see Wing Chun or Ving Tsun Romanized for the 詠春 characters. The other spellings for 春 that have appeared in the recent years, such as Tjun, Tzun, Tsjun, or Tchun are not to be found in any academic transliterations, but done by non-Chinese practitioners wanting to rebrand the art for themselves.

Although the Hong Kong Government adopted the Pinyin method for Romanizing Cantonese, which I find quite easy to understand because of my familiarity with Pinyin for Mandarin, I am not using it for the book since it would be too unfamiliar for English readers. For example, *c* is allocated for the *ts* sound. So 春 is spelled *ceon*. For the book, I will use the familiar spellings or use Yale or Pinyin (Jyutping in Cantonese) or my own transliteration—whichever I believe would be the easiest to pronounce.

ACKNOWLEDGMENTS

I'D LIKE TO THANK the many people who've one way or another contributed to the publication of this book—my *first* ever.

First and foremost, I thank my co-author, John Little, without whom my work would never have gone to print. It was through his encouragements, contacts, and experience that made it possible.

I'd also like to thank Skyhorse Publishing, Inc., for trusting and giving me, an unknown writer, the opportunity to present my work for publication.

I'd like to particularly thank Stephen Levin, MD, for not only giving me permission to use his material on biotensegrity found in Chapter Ten, "Structure: The Science of Architecture," but for also advising me on it.

I thank the great Grandmaster Ip Man (葉問) for sharing his art with his many fine students in Hong Kong, but in particular with Lok Yiu (駱耀), Moy Yat (梅逸) and Wong Shun Leung (黃淳梁). It was through the efforts of these men in teaching Wing Chun that the art eventually spread outside of Hong Kong and eventually came to my attention through certain students of these gentlemen, namely Winston Wan (雲), Wong Siu Leung (黃兆良) and Nelson Chan (陳就祥). These fine men are not only my teachers in the art of Wing Chun, but also my dear friends.

I thank my Wing Chun Sisook (師叔) Lester Lau (劉梅義), my Sihings (師 兄) Keene Low (劉志堅) and late Vasco Texiera, for helping me in my Wing Chun journey.

I thank my other teachers who contributed towards my development as a martial artist, such as my Judo teacher Hua Nan; my Taekwondo teacher, Park Jong Soo; my Wu Taiji (Tai Chi) teacher, Zhou Shifu; my Chen Taiji teacher, Lu Yong (呂勇); my Qigong teachers Catherine Kurz (藍麗鳳) and Luo Kangqi (骆康啟).

I thank my disciples worldwide, who had not only supported me in my Wing Chun career, but had also taught me to become a better teacher. I thank Jeeraphan (Yut) Kanchanaveera, Richy May, Jan Schmidt-Burback, Bart Cowling, Rapin (Ming) Rookbanyang, Suthep Srikureja, Andy Hall, Javed Khan, Marilyn Algava, Basheer Hatahet, Michel Interresse, Lam Vu, Michael Charles, Almoatasimballh Almizyen, Anthony Tan, Baard Wiliams, and Alessandro Cataldo.

I thank those who've invited me to their countries to teach them and/ or conduct seminars, such as Mehdi Hijaouy and Abdul Karim of Morocco; Rafael Avella i Riera of Spain; George Jonker, Russell Clark, and Renato Villareal of Australia; Niles Maxwell and Michael Helle of Germany; Ben Buchli of Switzerland; Eddie Hodemniac of Belgium; Zayid Jones, Omar Gamal, Nabil Adam, Abbas Rahman, and Andrew Kitchingham of New Zealand.

I'd like to thank my current students in Canada who stood by me through my hardships in the two years I've been here starting life anew. I especially thank David Forbes and David Miller who have stayed with me steadfastly since the beginning.

I thank my students who participated in the making of this book by modeling for the photographs. They are Isaac Boyes, James Hillman, David Miller, Joseph O'Donnell, Jiayu Zheng, and Angel Zheng.

I thank my three ex-wives, Teresa Wong, Somkhit Ratseeha, and Keaw Narinnon, and my three daughters—Yulin, Selene, and Acelin, for letting me take time away from home to pursue my passion of becoming a martial artist and teacher. None of them had ever made one single complaint.

And most importantly, I thank each and every member of my family for making me who I am. Without their support and influences, this book may never have come to be. I thank my late father, Mingshan (明善), for inspiring me to become a warrior from listening to his heroic adventures; my late mother, Yulien (玉蓮), for teaching me to be righteous; my sister, Helen (宝鈴), for rescuing the family out of a very insecure life in India; my brother John (尚中) for influencing me at a very young age on proper diet and exercises; my sister, Rose (鳳鈴), for teaching me to type as a youth, which has now led me to become a writer; and my brother, Jimmy (尚義), for physically fighting me, fighting for me, and fighting along side with me. We grew up in an environment where boys scuffled a lot to prove their manhood. Jimmy and I fought each other often. In my preteen years, the nearly four years age difference that Jimmy had over me made a big difference in our sizes, weight and height; so, I'd always lose my fight with him; however, that made me more determined, and wanting to take up skills that would turn the table around. So, when I finally enrolled in Judo, Taekwondo, and Wing Chun, I was fixed on becoming the best at them.

In life, we are affected by the environment and people around us. The results could be disastrous or favorable. However, whatever the outcome, it can be viewed positively as an experience gained in life, thus, making us who we are. I am who I am because of where I was, who I was with, and what had occurred. I thank all the people and events I've encountered in my life.

Danny Xuan (宣印生)

INDEX

About the Authors

DANNY XUAN

Danny Xuan has been a Wing Chun practitioner for over forty years. He travels internationally to instruct and has been featured in documentaries on the art produced by studios such as Warner Bros. Danny writes an instructional column for *Wing Chun Illustrated* magazine and currently resides in Ontario, Canada. His website provides unique insights into the art of Wing Chun.

JOHN LITTLE

John Little has been a martial arts practitioner for over thirty years, studying first in Karate and later training in Jeet Kune Do privately with Ted Wong, one of Bruce Lee's top students. He has written extensively on martial arts and produced several award-winning documentary films (*Wing Chun: The Art That Introduced Kung Fu To Bruce Lee*; *Bruce Lee: A Warrior's Journey*) for major studios such as Warner Bros. He is the author of over forty books on martial arts, fitness, bodybuilding, history and philosophy and was voted into the American Martial Arts Hall Of Fame.